WHAT YOU NEED TO KNOW ABOUT COMPLEXION PERFECTERS

THE CHEMISTRY BEHIND ACHIEVING BEST RESULTS WITH YOUR COSMETICS

HARMINDER GILL

authorHOUSE®

AuthorHouse™
1663 Liberty Drive
Bloomington, IN 47403
www.authorhouse.com
Phone: 1 (800) 839-8640

All information and data presented in this minibook is subject to change
without notice. Neither Author House nor its affiliates, employees, agents,
or authors shall be liable for any damage or injury caused by information
presented throughout the minibook. You understand and agree that the
material presented is for learning, research, and any acts carried out is
done at your own risk and discretion. You are solely responsible for all
outcomes based on your ability to use cosmetics in the right and proper
fashion. Please do check with a beauty consultant if you are ever in doubt.

Published by AuthorHouse 11/17/2016

ISBN: 978-1-5246-5110-7 (sc)
ISBN: 978-1-5246-5109-1 (e)

Print information available on the last page.

This book is printed on acid-free paper.

Table of Contents

Acknowledgements

I wish to acknowledge Author House for taking the time to publish this book. Thank you very much for the time and dedication to make this book possible. Special thank you to Ms. Christal Petrak, spa owner, beauty and skincare expert for her insight and wisdom.

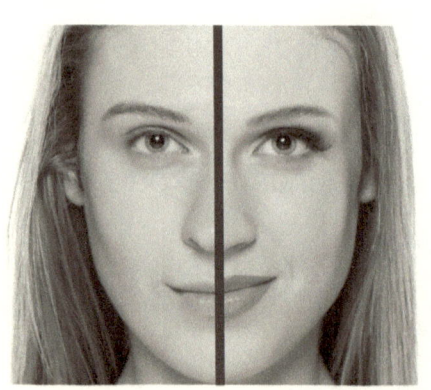

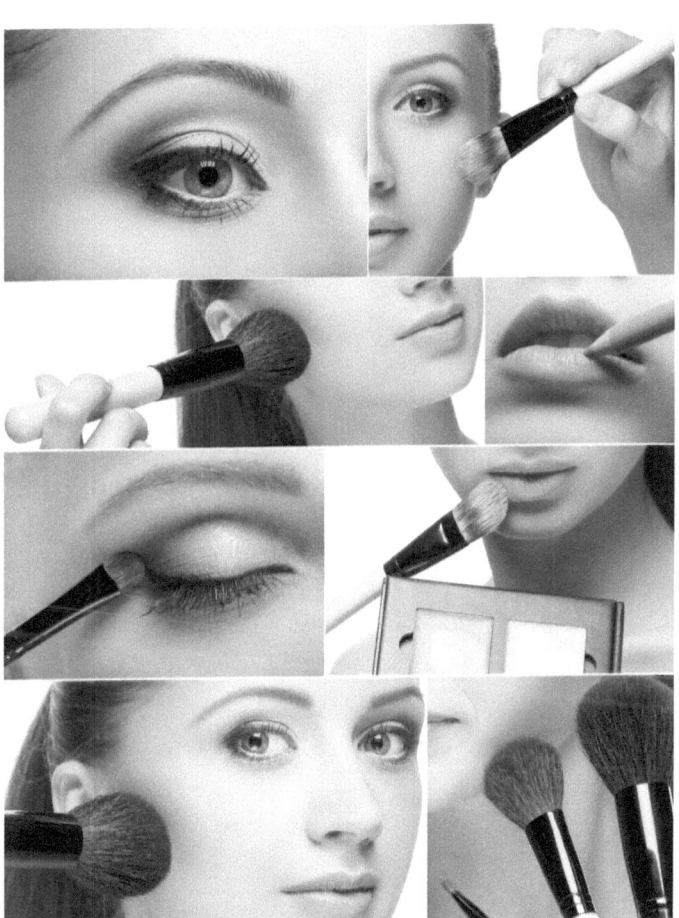

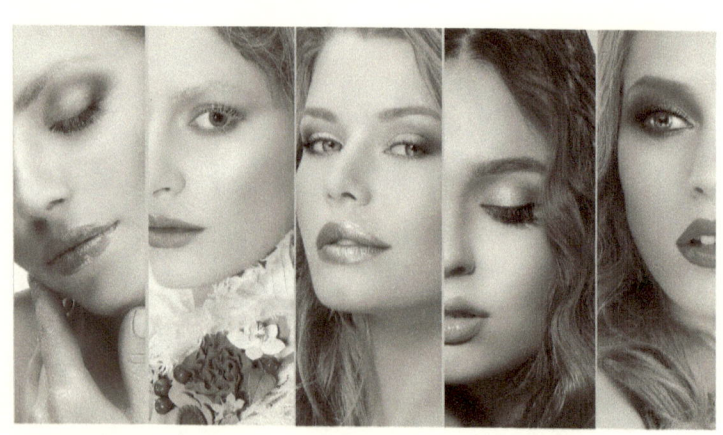

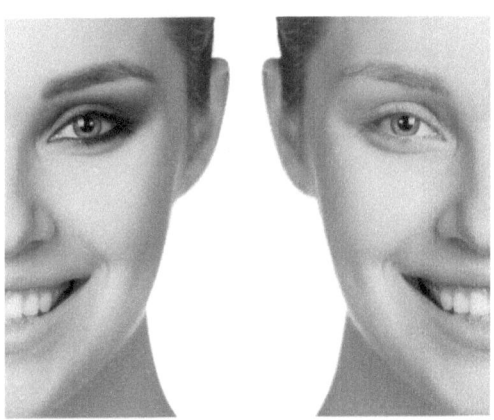

Chapter 1

Introduction

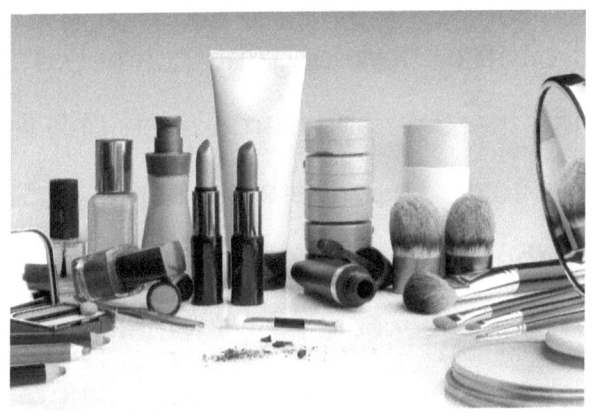

The purpose of cosmetic chemistry is to introduce the fundamental principles of cosmetic formulation. It is the intent of this minibook to provide a general science background and to have the reader learn more about cosmetics. Many women open their makeup bags and apply lipstick, mascara, eye shadow, foundations, concealers, and other kinds of make-up without knowing what they are putting on. Some women look for naturally made products, products that are hypoallerginic and oil free, how long the cosmetics last during the day, and some even only look at the color. Then there are some females who choose not to wear makeup because it is so time-consuming. Whether you wear makeup or not, it is important to know the pros and cons of makeup. All make-up consists of many natural ingredients as well as chemicals, and they need to be put on wisely for best results. We can think of a chemical as a basic substance. Understanding the chemistry of each of the cosmetics should help make a wise decision choosing the right product on the skin. Inflammation, premature aging, and hyperpigmentation are factors a lot of people are concerned about when it comes to taking care of their skin. Anti-aging or age management is what I'm also hoping the reader to get out of this minibook.

The purpose of chemicals in cosmetic products is to improve and refine the appearance of skin, lips, lashes, and other body and facial features. However, applying make-up is not that easy since some of it can cause serious adverse side effects. The first thing to do is to read and study the labels. The United States Food and Drug Administration makes it a requirement for cosmetic manufacturers to put labels on the listing ingredients in descending order of weight. Ingredients that contain less than one percent of make-up consist of fragrance or colorants. These are listed after the other ingredients. Make-up users need to be careful to reduce the chances of developing rashes, eye infections, acne, or other health related problems involving cosmetics.

Human Skin

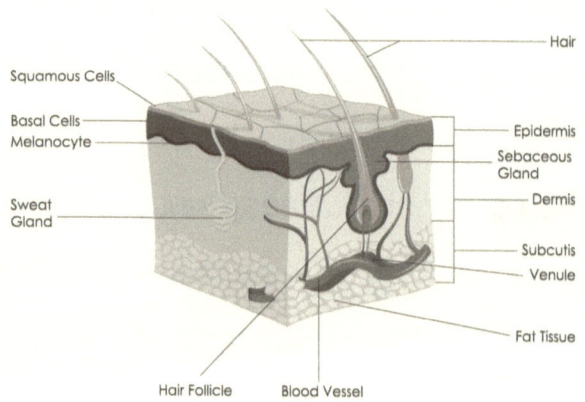

Consumers should not waste money on cosmetics that are expensive than those cosmetics that are less expensive if they are going to get the same results.

How do we define cosmetic chemistry? Cosmetic chemistry deals with changes that take place at the microscopic level. Very few understand what goes on at the microscopic level or the chemistry between elements, compounds, or molecules. In general, cosmetic chemistry can be defined as the study of the effects of raw materials and mixtures that can have on different parts of the human body. These include the hair, the skin, the nails, the lips, and other parts of the body.

Cosmetic scientists must always be professional and have high ethics when working in this field. If you are interested making or marketing make-up, hair products, nail polish, and the wide variety of cosmetic items, then you might want to consider choosing a career in cosmetic science. It would be good to continue to learn more about the fields of cosmetic science and the many associated careers offered in the job market.

If you are interested pursing a school in cosmetic science, then one must complete a bachelor's degree in a scientific field and score high on the Graduate Record Examination if you choose to pursue advanced degrees. Degree programs can be found in schools or even online. Some degree programs online may require classroom hours.

If you decide to go into occupations involving research and development, it will be a good idea to complete a bachelor's, master's, or doctoral degree in biological chemistry with an emphasis in cosmetic science. Typical cosmetic science classes include skin care raw materials and formulations, microtoxicity, perfumery, quality assurance, product development, color cosmetics, dermal pharmacology, polymer chemistry, and many other available classes. Marketing courses may include international marketing, marketing research, product and brand management, marketing strategies, and even sales advertising.

Possible career paths include odorant manufacturer, color specialist for a pigment, quality assurance, nutritional production formulations, chemical ingredient manufacturer, research and development, and many more positions are offered. There is a need for products to be tested and for businesses to discover and test brand new products. Some people may choose to go into research for pure scientific discovery. There is also sales and marketing careers in cosmetic science as well. Once research and development is done to make the product, the product then needs to be marketed and sold to the public. It is important to understand the materials used to create the product and to be able to describe them to the public. Job positions are expected to be best for those who have advanced degrees. There is a lot of strong competition for cosmetic science positions, but those who have knowledge of internet-based advertising should be able to be more competitive.

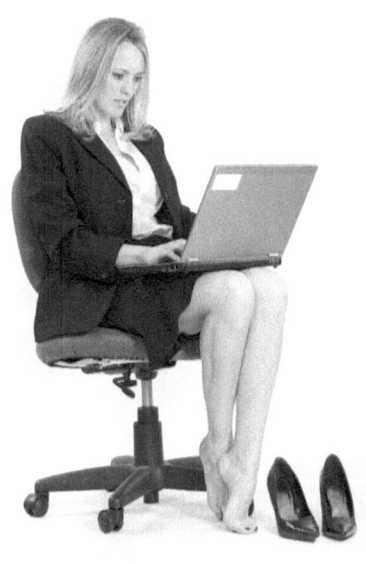

The beginning of the book was written to cover basic biological chemistry before proceeding to cosmetics. It is important to know the chemistry that takes place in solution to have a deeper understanding of cosmetics. Biomolecules are discussed to cover the fundamental structure of proteins and other larger molecules used in cosmetic chemistry research. Research is always being carried out throughout the world, and it could replace some of the content presented in this minibook in the future.

Regardless of the science course you took or if you have never seen topics covered in science, you will find that the microscopic world of science is different from the macroscopic world in which we live in. Both worlds are highly connected to each other. The science that takes place in the microscopic world greatly affects the science that takes place in the macroscopic world. Currently, we are in the twenty-first century, and at this day and age we have a stronger understanding of atoms, molecules, compounds, and reactions than we did almost one hundred years ago due to upgraded technology. But we still have many more questions that remain unanswered such as how and why some reactions take place and an accurate representation of most of the mechanisms that take place in reactions. A better understanding of these factors can help cosmetic scientists formulate even better products for many consumers.

The minibook then briefly talks about cosmetic beauty tips that might be helpful for long term. When using beauty products, keep the following information in mind. The shelf life of beauty products don't last very long. Concealers last up to twelve months. Eye shadows last up to three years. Facial cleansers last up to one year. Lip liners last up to three years. Lipsticks depending on the type will last up to one to four years. Makeup brushes made of natural fibers can last several years, but they need to be washed about every two to three months with a mild detergent.

Mascara can last up to four months. Makeup sponges should be washed on a weekly basis and then discarded on a monthly basis. Sponges have the ability to accumulate bacteria. Nail polish can last up to twelve months. If you sharpen the pencil eyeliner on a regular basis, the pencil liners will last for three years. Powder can last up to two years. Perfumes can last from three to five years starting when it was first produced. Furthermore, fragrances, however, have the ability to last longer.

Besides taking care of all the cosmetics you need to use, keep in mind the consumer still needs to take care of herself. It is good to stay young and reduce signs of aging by not eating too much, making love, keep learning a variety of things in life, reducing belly fat, eating more plant-rich foods, and drinking red wine as long as you are not allergic to plant-rich foods and red wine. Please do check with your doctor to see what would work best for you. Besides that let us now explore the microsopic world of the chemistry of cosmetics.

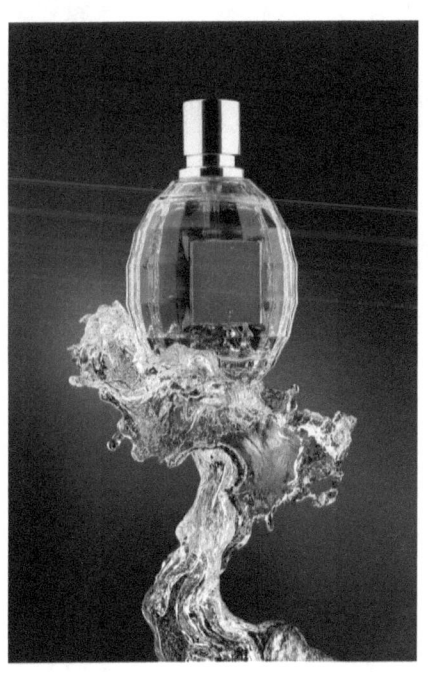

Chapter 2

Biomolecules

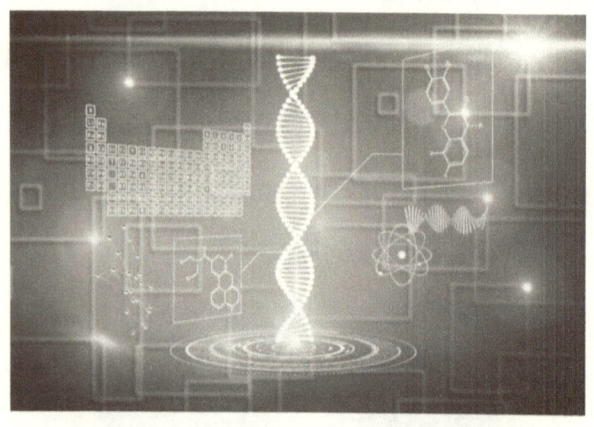

Body fat is important when taking care of ourselves especially when it comes time to take care of our skin. Body mass is made of protoplasm, extracellular fluid, bone, and adipose tissue. We can determine the amount of adipose tissue by measuring the whole-body density. The mass of the body is determined on land. The underwater body mass can be determined by submerging a person in water. Water helps support the body by giving it buoyancy. The underwater body mass is expected to be less. A higher amount of percentage of body fat makes a person more buoyant. It causes the underwater mass to be smaller. Fat has a lower density than the rest of the body. The difference between land mass and underwater mass is called buoyant force. This is used to determine body volume. Both mass and volume can be used to determine body density. Once the body density is determined, it can be compared to a chart that correlates the percentage of adipose tissue with body density.

Another way we can take care of our skin is through weight. The number of kilocalories that is needed in the daily diet for an adult depends both on sex and activity. If the amount of food intake exceeds energy output, then body weight for a person increases. The amount of food we take is regulated by the hunger center in the hypothalamus which is located in the brain. Regulating food intake is proportional to how much nutrients is stored in the body. If the nutrients are low, then a person feels hungry. If the nutrients are high, then a person does not want to eat anything. Weight reduction takes place when the amount of food intake is less than the output of energy. Muscular exercise is a good way to expend energy. Increasing daily exercise gives weight loss.

There are also certain elements essential for our skin. There are four elements that make up carbohydrates, fats, proteins, and deoxyribonucleic acid or DNA. These four elements are carbon, hydrogen, oxygen, and nitrogen. The majority of hydrogen and oxygen is found in water which is made up of 55-60% of the body mass. The following elements are essential to health: oxygen, carbon, hydrogen, nitrogen, calcium, phosphorus, potassium, sulfur, sodium, chlorine, magnesium, iron, fluorine, zinc, copper, and iodine. There are also important trace elements that is needed in the body. Even though they are required in extremely small amounts, without them they disrupt biological processes and cause illnesses.

Let us take a look at iron which has the chemical symbol Fe. The adult daily value for males is 10 mg, whereas for females it is 18 mg. Iron's role is the formation of hemoglobin and to help enzymes. If you do not get enough iron, deficiency symptoms include dry skin, spoon nails, anemia, and decreased hemoglobin. We can get plenty of iron in green leafy vegetables, 100% whole wheat breads, and cereals. The amount of copper intake for an adult should be around 2.0 to 5.0 mg. Copper is needed for enzyme systems, growth, and helping with the formation of red blood cells and collagen. Without enough copper, a person can get anemia, decreased white blood cell count, and bone demineralization. Dietary sources for copper include nuts, whole grains, and leafy green vegetables.

The adult intake for zinc is 15 mg. Zinc has a role in amino acid metabolism, energy production, enzyme systems, and collagen. If there is not enough zinc, there will be retarded bone formation, skin inflammation, a loss of smell and taste, and poor healing. Zinc can be found in 100% whole wheat grains. The adult intake for manganese should be between 2.5 - 5.0 mg. Manganese is necessary for enzyme systems, the formation of collagen, fat and carbohydrate metabolism, the central nervous system, and blood clotting. If there is not enough manganese there will be abnormal skeletal growth and the central nervous system will malfunction. Manganese can be found in 100% whole grains, wheat germs, legumes, figs, and pineapple.

The normal intake for iodine is 150 µg. Iodine is necessary for the activity of the thyroid gland. If there is not enough iodine, then a person can get hypothyroidism, goiter, or even cretinism. Iodine can be found in seafood and iodized salt. The normal intake for fluorine is 1.5 - 4.0 mg. Fluorine is necessary for the formation of teeth and it helps retain calcium in bones with aging. Without enough fluorine, a person can get dental cavities. Fluorine can be found in tea, fish, supplementary drops, and some areas with water.

Ions in body fluids are needed for physiological and metabolic functions which is also important for the skin. The sodium cation is outside the cell. It regulates and controls body fluids. Sodium is found in salt, cheese, and pickles. Too little sodium leads to hyponatremia, diarrhea, anxiety, circulatory failure, and a decrease in body fluid. Obtaining too much sodium gives hypernatremia, thirst, edema, and even little urine. The potassium cation is found inside the cell. Potassium regulates body fluids and cellular functions. Potassium is found in bananas, milk, orange juice, prunes, and potatoes. If we do not get enough potassium, we can develop hypokalemia, muscle weakness, lethargy, and neurological impulses not working. If we get too much potassium then we could get hyperkalemia, irritability, nausea, little urine, and even cardiac arrest.

Calcium cations are found outside the cells. About 90% of calcium in the body in bone is either $Ca_3(PO_4)_2$ or $CaCO_3$. Calcium is a major cation of bone and muscle smoothant. We can get plenty of calcium from milk, cheese, yogurt, greens, and spinach. Too little calcium intake results in hypocalcemia, tingling fingertips, osteoporosis, and muscle cramps. Too much calcium results in hypercalcemia, kidney stones, relaxed muscles, and deep bone pain. Magnesium cations are found outside the cell. About 70% of magnesium in the body is bone structure. Magnesium is essential for certain enzymes, muscles, and nerve control. Magnesium can be found in nuts and whole grains. Too little magnesium results in slow pulse, tremors, disorientation, and hypertension. Too much magnesium results in drowsiness. The chlorine anion is also found outside the cell. It is found in gastric juice and regulation of body fluids. The chloride anion can be found in salt. Too little and too much of the chloride anion gives the same effects as the sodium cation.

The health of our teeth also has a profound effect on the skin. Bone structure is made up of two parts. It is made of a solid mineral and a second phase made of collagen proteins. The mineral substance is called hydroxyapatite. It is a solid formed from calcium ions, phosphate ions, and hydroxide ions. The material is deposited on collagen to form calcium hydroxyapatite. The chemical structure is $Ca_{10}(PO_4)_6(OH)_2$. Bone material is always being absorbed and formed. After 40 years old, it is possible for more bone material to be lost than formed. It is a condition called osteoporosis. Reduction of bone mass takes places faster in women than in men. Rate of reduction is different in different parts of the skeleton. Bone mass can be reduced as much as 50% from a period of 30 - 40 years. People over 35 years old, especially women, take a daily calcium supplement in their diet.

A lot of people taking care of their skin are also concerned about using hot packs and cold packs. Cold packs can be used to reduce swelling when there is an injury. It can reduce heat from inflammation, or it can decrease capillary size to lesson hemorrhaging. Cold packs contain ammonium nitrate (NH_4NO_3) which is separated from a compartment of water. The pack can be activated when it is squeezed hard enough to break the walls between compartments. Ammonium nitrate then mixes with the water. The process is endothermic which means it absorbs energy. Ammonium nitrate dissolves and absorbs 6.3 kcal of heat from water. Temperature drops and the pack itself becomes cold. Hot packs, however, are used to relax muscles. They lessen aches and cramps. They also increase circulation by expanding capillary size. Hot packs contain the salt calcium chloride ($CaCl_2$). Dissolving this salt in water is exothermic and releases 18 kcal per mole. The temperature rises and then becomes hot.

Taking care of our skin also involves us to understand the amount of water in our body. Average adults contain about 60% water by weight. The average infant contains about 75% water by weight. There is about 60% of the body's water that is contained within the cells as intracellular fluids. The other 40% is made up of extracellular fluids. These include interstitial fluids in tissue and plasma found in blood. The external fluids carry nutrients and waste materials between both cells and the circulatory system. Just about every day we lose 1,500 ml to 3,000 ml of water from our kidneys as urine, from the skin as perspiration, from the lungs being exhaled, and from the gastrointestinal tract. Dehydration can happen to an adult if there is a 10% net loss of total body fluid. Losing 20% of fluid can also be fatal. Infants can suffer dehydration with a 5-10% loss of body fluid. Water needs to be continuously replaced by liquids and foods in the diet. They also need to be replaced by metabolic processes that make water in the cells of the body.

Let us take a look at alpha hydroxy acids or AHAs. They are naturally occuring carboxylic acids, and they are found in fruits, milk, and sugarcane. High concentrations of AHAs have been used to remove acne scars, reduce irregular pigmentation, and age spots. Lower concentrations of AHAs are added to skin care products for smoothing fine lines, improving the texture of the skin, and to clean pores. Glycolic acid and lactic acid are popular. Keep in mind that products that contain AHAs increase the sensitivity of the skin to both sun and ultraviolet radiation. Sunscrean with a sun protection factor or SPF of at least 15 can be used when treating the skin that have products which include AHAs. Products that have AHAs at concentrations under 10% and pH values larger than 3.5 are normally considered safe. But the Food and Drug Administration have reported AHAs to have caused skin irritation such as blisters, rashes, and discoloration of the skin. Keep in mind the FDA is not required to have product safety reports from cosmatic manufacturers. But they do their best to market safe products. The FDA recommends to test any product containing AHAs on small areas of the skin before applying it to larger areas of the skin. Sources of alpha hydroxy acids include glycolic acid which is from sugarcane or sugarbeet, lactic acid from sour milk, tartaric acid from grapes, malic acid from apples or grapes, citric acid from citrus fruits such as lemon, oranges, and grapefruit.

Cell membranes separates the contents of a cell from the exterior of the environment. It also contains structures that communicate with other cells. The synthesis of proteins takes place inside cells. Proteins are considered to be linear polymers. They can be synthesized from twenty different standard alpha amino acids by condensation to form peptide bonds. The amino groups have carboxyl groups with a pK near 2.2 whereas the amino group have a pK near 9.4 attached to the alpha carbon. Alpha amino acids are zwitterionic compounds in their physiological pH range.

Biogenic Amino Acids (22 formulas)

There are various amino acids that are classified according to their polarities of their side chains. The side chains are also substituents to the alpha carbon atom. Nonpolar amino acids include glycine, alanine, valine, leucine, isoleucine, phenylalanine, tryptophan, and methionine. Proline is a nonpolar secondary amino acid. Amino acids that have uncharged polar side chains include serine, threonine, asparagine, glutamine, tyrosine, and cysteine. Amino Acids that have charged polar side chains include lysine, arginine, histidine, aspartic acid, and glutamic acid.

Side chains of amino acids contain acid-base groups which give rise to the properties of proteins that depend on pH. Alpha carbon atoms of the alpha amino acids contain four different substituents and are called chiral centers. Glycine is an exception, and it is considered to be achiral. Derivatives of amino acids can also be used to make proteins.

There are only 10 amino acids that can be synthesized in the body. The other 10 amino acids are considered to be essential amino acids that can't be synthesized and must be obtained from proteins in the diet. Ten of the essential amino acids include arginine, histidine, isoleucine, leucine, lysine, methionine, phenylalanine, threonine, tryptophan, and valine. The amino acids arginine and histidine are required in diets for children and not adults. Complete proteins contain all of the essential amino acids. They are found in animal products such as eggs, milk, fish, meat, and poultry. Gelatin and plant proteins are found in grains, beans, and nuts. They are considered to be incomplete proteins since they are deficient in one or more essential amino acids. Diets that consume plant foods for protein must contain other protein sources to obtain all of the essential amino acids. Rice and beans are complementary protein sources. Beans contain lysine which is not found in rice. Rice contains methionine and tryptophan which is not enough found in beans.

Protein function is related to protein structure. When we think of structure we think of the three-dimensional relationships between the protein's individal atoms. Proteins can be described based on four levels of organization. The primary structure of a protein is the amino acid sequence of the polypeptide chains. The secondary structure is viewed as the spatial arrangement of the polypeptide's backbone atoms. The conformations of the side chains are not important. The tertiary structure is described as the three-dimensional structure of the polypeptide itself. Proteins can also be made up of two or more polypeptide chains. These polypeptide chains are referred to as subunits which contain noncovalent interactions and some of these chains contain disulfide bonds. The quaternary structure of a protein refers to how the spatial arrangement of the subunits are located.

There are different types of proteins. Fibrous proteins, for example, can be correlated with structure. Keratin is the main component of hair and nails that form protofibrils and consist of two pairs of alpha helices that are twisted together in a left-hand coil. The flexibility of keratin decreases as disulfide bond cross-links between protofibrils increases. Keratin is also found in skin and wool. Silk fibroin has the ability to form flexible, but the inextensive fibers are of great strength. It has a semicrystalline array of antiparallel beta sheets where layers of glycine side chains alternate with layers with alanine and serine side chains.

Collagen is the main protein component of connective tissue. Collagen is found in tendons and cartilage. Every third residue is glycine. The other amino acids are proline and hydroxyproline. Collagen, therefore, forms a triple helical structure with strong tensile strength. Collagen molecules have the ability to aggregate to form fibrils. These fibrils are covalently cross-linked by derivative groups of histidine and lysine. Elastin have elastic properties and form a three-dimensional network of fibers that have no regular structure. The polypeptide strands are cross-linked just like collagen.

Carbohydrates are another abundant class of molecules. The basic unit of carbohydrates are monosaccharides. Examples of monosaccharides include glyceraldehyde, erythrose, threose, ribose, arabinose, xylose, lyxose, allose, altrose, glucose, mannose, gulose, idose, galactose, and talose. Two monosaccharides joined together is called a disaccharide. Several monosaccharides joined together forms a polysaccharide.

Another class of molecules are fatty acids. Fatty acids are considered to be long chain carboxylic acids. They can have one or more double bonds that are usually cis. The anions are considered to be amphiphilic and form micelles in water.

Fatty acids usually don't occur in nature but are components of lipids. Triacylglycerols are also called neutral fats and fall under the class called lipids. They are nonpolar molecules that are usually nonsoluble in aqueous solutions.

Carbohydrates, proteins, and lipids are similar since they are sources of energy. Unlike carbohydrates, proteins and lipids are similar and contain monomers to make polymers. Unlike lipids, carbohydrates and proteins make up a larger group of molecules called macromolecules. Unlike proteins, carbohydrates and lipids are macronutrients. Proteins and carbohydrates differ slightly based on their chemical composition and dietary requirements. Proteins and lipids also differ from each other. Proteins are building blocks of energy that is needed by the body.

They make and repair hair, muscles, etc. Lipids are considered to be fats. They help by insulating the body. Carbohydrates and lipids also differ from each other by the fact that lipids contain nitrogen and sulfur with smaller constituents.

Enzymes are another class of biological molecules. They are very specific and bind their subtrates through both geometric and physical complementary interactions. This allows enzymes to be absolutely stereospecific when it comes to binding substrates and also for catalyzing reactions. Enzymes have the ability to vary their structure for geometric specificity. They can be highly specific whereas other substrates can bind a wide range of substrates and catalyze many kinds of reactions.

Vitamins are organic molecules that are needed for both health and growth. Fat-soluble vitamins include Vitamin A, Vitamin D, Vitamin E, and Vitamin K. Vitamin A is needed for the formation of visual pigments and for epithelial cells to develop. Vitamin D is needed for absorption of calcium and phosphate. Calcium and phosphate get deposited on the bone. Vitamin E is considered to be an antioxidant. It prevents the oxidation of Vitamin A and unsaturated fatty acids. Vitamin K is needed for the synthesis of prothrombin used for blood clotting.

Glycerol or glycerin is also called 1,2,3-Propanetriol. It is a trihydroxy alcohol which is a viscous liquid obtained from oils and fats when soaps are made. The presence of several hydroxyl groups make it strongly attracted to water. This feature makes glycerol good to use as a skin softener in products such as liquid soaps, skin lotions, shaving creams, and even in cosmetics. Exposure of formaldehyde fumes tends to irritate the nose, eyes, upper respiratory tract, headaches, dizziness, general fatigue, and even cause skin rashes. Acetone is used as nail polish remover, but it should be used carefully since it is flammable.

Oil of winter green is also considered to be methyl salicylate. It has a spearmint odor and flavor. It passes through the skin, and it is used in skin ointments where it can act as a counterirritant which produces heat to soothe sore muscles. Propyl acetate gives the odor of pears. Pentyl acetate gives the odor of bananas. Octyl acetate gives the odor of oranges. Ethyl butyrate gives the odor of pineapples. Pentyl butyrate gives the odor of apricots.

Saturated fatty acids such as lauric acid is found in coconut, myristic acid is found in nutmeg, palmitic acid is found in palm, and stearic acid is found in animal fat. Monounsaturated fatty acids such as palmitoleic acid is found in butter whereas oleic acid is found in olives and corn. Polyunsaturated fatty acids such as linoleic acid is found in soybean, safflower, and sunflower, and linolenic acid is found in corn.

Oleic (octadecenoic) acid

Ricinoleic (hydroxyoctadecanoic) acid

Erucic (docosenoic acid)

Linoleic (octadecadienoic acid)

Linolenic (octadecatrienoic acid)

Arachidonic (eicosatetraenoic acid)

Clupanodonic (docosanpentaenoic) acid

Chapter 3

Ingredients

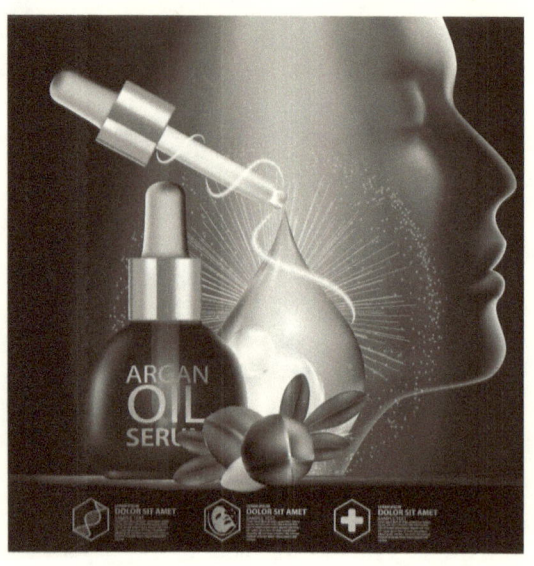

A primer is considered a cream or lotion that is applied before putting on another cosmetic. This helps improve coverage and makes the amount of time the cosmetic to last longer on the face. Examples of cosmetic primers include foundation primers, eyelid primers, lip primers, and mascara primers. Foundation primers can work like a moisturizer. It can absorb oil with salicylic acid or help create a less oily appearance. It helps make the foundation to be smooth. Some of these foundation primers contain antioxidants (A, C, and E). Some of these primers also contain grape seed extract and green tea extract. There are two types of foundation primers. These include water-based and silicon-based. They contain the ingredients cyclomethicone and dimethicone. Note that some of these primers don't contain preservatives, oil, or fragrance. Some of them can have sun protection factor and even improve skin tone. Foundation primers can also be mineral-based primers that contain mica and silica. Eyelid or eye shadow primer evens out the color of the lid and the area near the upper eye. It could reduce oiliness and add shimmer. These primers help smoothen the application of eye shadow and stop it from building up in eyelid creases. Eyelid primers are put on the eyelid and the lower eye area before eye shadow is applied. The color of the eye shadow is intensified, and it helps them from smearing by the reduction of oiliness of the lids. Eye shadow primers can also work for eyeliners and eye shadow bases. Other primers include mascara primer. Some of the mascara primers are colorless. It thickens and lengthens the lashes before mascara is applied. The lashes last longer when primers are used. Lip primers smoothen the lips and improve the appearance when lipstick is applied. It is recommended lip gloss be used to exfoliate the lips before applying the lip primer. Color lasts longer and makes sure the lipstick does not smear and migrate into the lines around the lips. The bottom line is foundation primers allow the foundation to stay on during hot weather. They help prevent the skin from absorbing talc and pigment from the foundation. It also prevents talc from drawing oil from the skin. To soothe and refreshen the skin, botanicals such as lavender, grape, kiwi, rose, jasmine, orange, and aloe extracts are added and used in the foundation process.

Lipstick consist of different waxes, oils, emollients, and pigments. Lipstick is used to put color on, to add texture, and to protect the female's lips. Waxes give the structure of solid lipstick. Waxes can be made from beeswax, ozokerite, and candelilla wax. Beeswax is made up of esters of straight-chain monohydric alcohols that have even-numbered carbon chains from C24 to C36. They also have straight-chain acids that have even numbers of carbon atoms up to C36. Caranuba wax comes from the pores of Brazilian wax palm tree leaves. Carnauba wax has a high melting point, and it also provides the strength of the lipstick. Candilla wax comes from the candilla plant produced in Mexico. The plants are placed in boiling water mixed with sulfuric acid which skims the wax off that goes to the surface. Oils and fats are also found in lipsticks, pigments, and oils. These include olive oil, mineral oil, cocoa butter, lanolin, and petrolatum. Most of the lipsticks in the United States contain pig fat or castor oil.

These give a strong and shiny look when it dries up after use. But if large amounts of castor oil are consumed, it could cause the need to urinate. Moisturizers such as Vitamin E, aloe vera, collagen, amino acids, and sun screen are also put in lipstick. These ingredients keep the lips soft, moisturized, and protected. The color of lipsticks comes from a variety of pigments and lake dyes. These include bromo acid, D & C Red No. 21, Calcium Lake (D & C Red 7 and D & C Red 34), and D & C Orange No. 17. Mixing colorless titanium dioxide and red shades gives pink lipsticks. Both organic and inorganic pigments are present. Matte lipsticks have more filling agents such as silica, but they do not have a lot of emollients. Crème lipsticks have more waxes than oils. Sheer and long-lasting lipstick has a lot of oil. Long lasting lipstick has silicone oil. This seals the colors to the person's lips. Glossy lipstick has more oil and provides a shiny finish to the lips. Lipstick that looks shimmery has mica, silica, fish scales, and pearl particles.   Let us look at the chemistry of lipstick. The pigments in lipstick can be separated using thin layer chromatography. The mobile phase can vary depending on the kind of pigment. Lipsticks are considered to be soluble in toluene. Normally, toluene is used as the mobile phase. Once the separation process is complete, a chromatogram shows the different pigments that compose the lipstick. Lipstick can be made from grinding and heating specific ingredients. Waxes that are heated are added to the mixture. Oils and lanolin are also added. Then the hot mixture is poured onto a metal mold. The mixture is then cooled so the lipstick can harden. After the lipstick is hardened, it is heated in a flame for less than a second to give a shiny appearance.

Concealers are considered to be color correctors. The purpose of concealers is to mask dark circles, age spots, and blemishes that are seen on the skin. It is thicker than foundation, and it has different pigments. It does this by blending around the skin. Concealers are applied after the primer and before the foundation on the face. Using concealers and foundations make the skin more even toned based on its color. Concealers have more pigments in them. It can be found in the liquid or solid form. Foundation is normally put on larger areas. Women can use concealers by itself or with foundations. Concealers are available from the lightest and deepest shades. Women have a tendency to choose shades lighter than their skin tone to hide blemishes and dark circles under the eye. Some of the colors give the natural skin tone, while others are used to contrast with a blemish. Concealers that have yellow undertones hide dark circles. The colors green and blue counteracts red patches on the skin-like pimples, broken veins, or rosacea. Concealers that are purple make the complexions look brighter. Colored concealers are applied a little bit beneath a concealer or foundation to match the female's skin tone. Concealers that are skinned toned are sufficient at covering up imperfections. Common concealer ingredients include talc, macadamia oil, and ground mica. Titanium dioxide and shea butter is also found in many concealers. Talc and titanium oxide could irritate the lungs if someone breathes into them. Some people are also allergic or could get skin irritation from macadamia oil, mica, and shea butter. Normally, other kinds of minerals and vitamins become mixed to make the final product. Talc gives a nice shimmer. Macadamia oil has a slight odor, but it is covered up with other ingredients. Ground mica reduces the appearance of wrinkles and other blemishes. Mica also protects the skin by blocking rays from the sun. Titanium dioxide protects us from the sun. It forms a barrier between the skin and harmful rays.

Foundation is considered to be a skin colored cosmetic put on the face to make a uniform color to hide flaws and to change the skin tone. Both coverage and formulation is used in foundation, opacity of makeup, transparency, and contains a small amount of pigment. It does not hide discolorations on the skin. It minimizes contrast between discoloration and skin tone. Light coverage covers blotchiness, but it does not cover freckles. Medium coverage can cover freckles, discolorations, and blotchiness. Full coverage is the most opaque. It is used to cover birthmarks, hyperpigmentation, and sears. Formulation has to do with ingredients blended together. Oil and emollient formulations consist of oil and emollient. Sheer coverage is pigment added to it. The texture is both thick and dense. Oil-based shakers can be applied to the skin with a texture that is smooth.

Liquid foundation works well around the eye. Alcohol-based formulations contain water and denatured alcohol as a base with pigment added to it. They don't clog pores and provides a sheerest coverage. Powder-based formulations uses powder mainly talc as one of the ingredients. Pigments, emollients, skin adhesion agents, and binding agents are added to the formula. Mineral makeup refers to foundation as loose powder. Common minerals include mica, bismuth oxychloride, titanium dioxide, or zinc oxide. Water-based formulations with emulsifiers formed a creamy liquid giving medium coverage. Water-based cream has a creamy texture. Water-based oil-free products contain an emollient ester or fatty alcohol, and it has a mattifying agent called clay. The oil-free mixtures are thick and heavy. Water-based transfer-resistant uses a polymer to give a matte finish. Silicon-based formulations contain silicone or a mixture of water and silicone. Normally, dimethicone and polysiloxane are used. Volatile silicones are also used. Silicone gives lubrication and viscosity to be put on the skin more evenly.

Face powder is powder put on the face. It sets a foundation ready for makeup to be applied. Two types of face powder include translucent sheer and pigmented powder. Some pigmented facial powders are worn alone that has no base foundation. Powder gives the face a more even appearance. Some powders also have sunscreen that reduces skin damage from sunlight and stress from the environment. Loose powder applied gives a uniform distribution. There are many colors of face powder and several types of it. Talc or baby powder is considered to be an absorbent and gives the tone of the skin. Face powder needs to be chosen carefully to match the tone of the skin.

Blush is also known as blusher or rouge. Women use blush to redden the cheeks to give a youthful appearance. It also emphasizes the cheekbones. Blush is made up of red talcum powder applied with a brush on the cheek. The coloring contains either the substance of safflor or carmine in ammonium hydroxide and rose water mixed with rose oil. Schnouda is also considered to be rouge. The mixture is colorless and contains Alloxan and cold cream. The purpose of bronze is to darken the complexion. You have to choose one based on skin tone. It should be two shades darker than your skin tone. It is best to use specialized bronzer brushes. Bronzer is added after the concealer and foundation has been put on.

Mascara is used to enhance the eyes. It could darken, thicken, and lengthen the eyelashes. It can be in the form of a liquid, cake, or cream. They contain the basic components of pigments, oils, waxes, and preservatives. The pigment for black mascara is carbon black. Brown mascaras use iron oxides. Some of them contain the pigment ultramarine blue. Specific oils such as mineral oil, linseed oil, castor oil, eucalyptus oil, lanolin, turpentine oil, and sesame oil is used. Paraffin wax, carnauba wax, and beeswax are common waxes found in mascara. The effects of mascara depend on the ingredients. An effect could be if the mascara is water resistant or not. Water-resistant mascaras have nonpolar substances such as dodecane. Non water-resistant mascaras have ingredients that are water-soluble. Mascaras that lengthen or curl eyelashes contain nylon or rayon microfibers. Ceresin, gum tragecanth, and methylcellulose are added to mascara to act as stiffeners. Proper disposal of mascara should be done after three months. If there is ever a bad odor of mascara, it should be disposed of properly. Mascara can grow bacteria so one should be careful. It is rare but possible that old mascara can cause eye infection or conjunctivitis, swollen eyelids, and stys. Swollen eyelids and stys are considered to be allergic reactions. The allergic reactions are normally due to the methylparaben, aluminum powder, ceteareth-20, butylparaben, or benzyl alcohol.

Let us take a look at the ingredient namely color. Make-up products give color and consistency. We think of red lips, shadowy eyelids, and puffy cheeks. A wide variety of colors are made on make-up racks. Many cosmetic chemists come up with dyes and pigments from many different compounds. Examples used to add color to our faces include coal tar, chromium oxide, aluminum powder, iron oxide, manganese, and mica flakes. Beet powder comes from plants. Pigments and dyes derived from animals include carmine which is a crimson pigment made from dried bodies of cochineal insect. Common coloring agents are the coal tar colors. Coal tar is sticky, and it is a black liquid made by heating bituminous coal in large ovens where air is absent. The colors of coal tar are made from ring-shaped aromatic hydrocarbons that are purified from the tar itself. These coal tar colors are the only makeup ingredients the FDA uses for safe testing of final products. Unfortunately, many of these compounds have been slow to cause cancer when injected into experimental rodents. Some of the coal tar colors are banned while some of them are approved. Once they pass safety tests, they are either given the designation FD & C (Food, Drugs, or Cosmetics) that means the color is safe for both internal and external uses. If the designation is D & C or Ext D & C then the compound is safe for external uses. Coloring agents such as D & C or Ext. D & C should not be applied where they are absorbed such as close to the eyes and on the lips which could cause blindness. Females who spread face foundation for their lips or eyelids before using lipstick or eye shadow should pay attention to the information provided on labels. Sometimes coal tar dyes can make or cause allergic or irritant reactions like rashes or inflammation. Yellow and red colors pose the problems.

Again, we can think of color coming from pigments and dyes. The compound titanium dioxide is considered to be a white pigment. Iron oxides can range in color from yellow, red, brown, and black. Mixing inorganic oxides and fillers makes face powders. Fillers are considered to be inert materials such as kaolin, talc, silica, and mica that are used to extend and develop colors. Mixing more ingredients such as oils and zinc stearate, and then pressing the mixture into pans make pressed powders such as eye shadows and blushers. Eye shadows and lipsticks contain pigments called pearls. The pearls tend to sparkle and reflect light to produce different kinds of colors. To prepare them, one precipitates a thin layer of color on mica that has thin platelets. If you vary the thickness of the color deposited, the angle of light changes, and it is refracted through the composite which then gives different colors. Organic pigments are also used to add color to lipsticks and eye shadows. If the organic compound is precipitated on a substrate, we call them laker pigments. We use the term lake to refer to the precipitating of an organic salt on a metal substrate. These are called D & C (drug and cosmetic) and FD & C (food, drug, and cosmetic) colors. Some of the dyes are soluble, and some of them are insoluble. Dyes give tints for lotions, oils, and shampoos.

Speaking of color, hair coloring products have the ability to mask or remove gray in the hair. Hair-coloring products react with protons in hair. These kind of products give a black-colored compound to cover up the gray in the hair. Hair-coloring products contain lead acetate, $Pb(O_2CH_3)_2$, which is soluble in aqueous solution. A reaction occurs between the Pb^{2+} aqueous cation and the sulfur atoms in cysteine and methionine that is also present in amino acids found in hair. The product of the reaction is lead(II) sulfide, PbS, which is insoluble.

Developing colors that seem attractive can be a challenge for chemists. Finding a way to make these colors stay on the face for many hours can also be difficult especially through times of perspiration, eating, or drinking. Make-up consists of another major ingredient class called bases. Almost every kind of makeup requires an oily mixture, which is considered a base to hold the colors together in a tube. This helps the colors stay on the face. The bases discussed have to do with manufacturing. The kind of base that is supposed to be used will depend on where it is supposed to be applied. Lipsticks consist of half of its weight by a thick insoluble mixture of waxes and castor bean oil. This does not dissolve when a female licks her lips or even drinks water. The lipstick base has to match the chemical properties of the ingredients in oil with wax. The oil found in the lipstick makes it thick and sticky so that the color stays on the lips. The waxes are considered to be thixotropic which means the waxes become fluid when stirred. They become thixotropic so the lipstick keeps its shape and so it does not smear or melt when heated.

Lipsticks also consist of esters. These are slippery chemical compounds. They are made by reactions between alcohols and acids. Esters make the lipstick shine and make dry oil and wax mixture smooth on the lips. Mascara, likewise, consist of heavy bases like paraffin and carnauba wax. They keep lash-darkening pigments stick to the eyelashes by water and tears. They also thicken and separate the lashes. Eye shadow, blush, and some powdery products stick together by lighter bases such as mineral oil. Most of the bases used for face foundation consist of mineral oil and water. The mixture of water and mineral oil gives an emulsion where tiny drops of a liquid are suspended in the second liquid. To help them stay together, emulsifying agents such as sodium stearate are added to make a creamy mixture.

Other bases include isopropyl lanolate or wool alcohol, myristyl lactate, and octyl hyroxystearate. These nontoxic compounds are called fatty esters. What is nice about bases is they cause very few allergic reactions. Lanolin products come from sheep's wool. Beeswax more likely does so too. Oils and waxes in makeup can cause acne for teenagers and young women. These greasy compounds give whiteheads, blackheads, and pimples because they can clog skin pores. Females who are prone to acne should carefully choose cosmetics that are both water soluble and free of oil.

Bulking agents are important ingredients in products that require even coverage like face powder and eye shadow. Examples of bulking agents include talc or French chalk, which is a powder, made from the mineral magnesium silicate. Talc is used in makeup because it absorbs perspiration. It also has a smooth and slippery texture. This helps make cosmetics easier to apply. You should never inhale deeply when using products containing talc like face powders, eye shadows, and powder blush. If you keep inhaling talc, you can develop lung problems. Other bulking agents such as silk powder can be added to eye shadow. Nylon and silk fibers can also be added to mascara. Be careful when using these products because silk powder triggers severe allergic reactions.

Waxes make up long chain esters that remain as solids at room temperature. Waxes are used in cosmetics. Specific waxes include beeswax, candelilla, carnauba, paraffin, and polyethylene. Waxes are found in lip balms and sticks. Waxes work by being structuring agents, and it makes the stick rigid enough to stand on its own. It also forms properties involving barriers. If you combine waxes with unique properties like brittleness, high shine, and flexibility, then the best cosmetic performance can be achieved. Waxes can also be combined with compatible oils to achieve softness. Turbidity and the separation of materials mixed together above their melting points determine compatibility. Waxes have been found to be useful for hand creams and mascara emulsions for thickening and waterproof properties.

Mixing wax with thin lotion, a thick cream is formed. A lot of the thickeners are considered to be polymers. Cellulose, for example, is considered to be a polymer of repeating D-glucose units. Cellulose tends to swell in hot water making a gel network. Carpool is a polyacrylic acid. It swells when it is neutralized. Bentone clays also swell when opened up through mechanical sheer. Carrageenan, pectin, and locust beam gum are also examples of cosmetic thickeners. Active ingredients are materials that work within the skin or help to protect the skin. An example is fruit acids. Fruit acids are also called alpha hydroxy acids or AHAs. They penetrate the skin where they increase the making of collagen, elastin, and intracellular substances that help improve the appearance of the skin. Many cosmetic active ingredients lighten, tighten, and make the skin firm. Active ingredients can also be used to suppress perspiration such as aluminum chlorohydrate. Other active ingredients include salicylic acid and benzoyl peroxide because of their ability to fight off acne. Petrolatum and dimethicone are also active ingredients to help protect the skin.

The purpose of sunscreens is to filter out most of the sun's burning rays. Many consumers are concerned about skin cancer and skin-damaging effects due to excessive exposure of the sun and harmful ultraviolet light. Compounds such as oxybenzone and dioxybenzone can also be used to carry this effect but the consumer should be careful, however, because these compounds can cause allergic reactions.

The point is that sunscreens protect the skin from ultraviolet radiation. Ultraviolet radiation with wavelengths 290 nm and 400 nm damage the skin. They have the ability to absorb or reflect wavelengths. The compound para (PABA) can be screened out. Sunscreen has the reflect damaging sun-protection factor or SPF. If you use sunscreen that has an SPF of 15 that means you will be able to be in the sun fifteen times longer than if left unprotected. Sunscreens can include octyl methoxycinnamate, octyl salcitate, titanium dioxide, and avobenzone. They are classified either as UVA or UVB sunscreens that depend on the wavelengths they absorb. Benzophenone-4 is considered to be a water-soluble UV filter. It used to protect the color of cosmetics.

Let us take a look at biological reactions involving UV light. Life depends on sunlight. But being exposed to a lot of sunlight damages the effects of living cells. Too much exposure can cause death. Light energy such as ultraviolet excites electrons and could lead to unwanted side effects on the skin. Damaging effects on sunlight include sunburn, wrinkling, premature aging of the skin, inflammation of the eyes, possibly cataracts, and even changes in DNA of cells which leads to skin cancers.

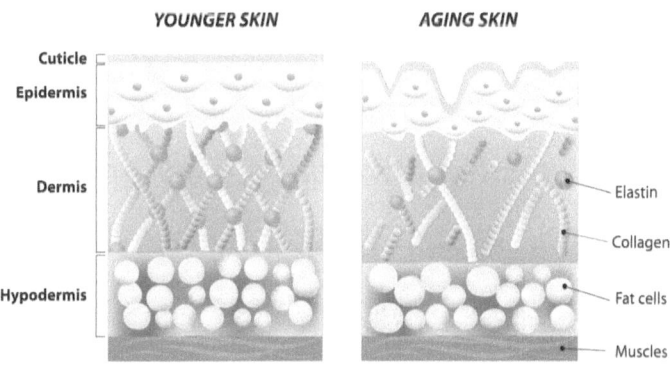

The consumer should be careful of acni medications such as Retin-A and Accutane. Other drugs to watch out for are diuretics, antibotics, sulfonamides, and estrogen which can also make the skin sensitive to light. Skin cancer has become common. DNA is damaged in exposed areas of the skin which causes mutations. Cells lose their ability to direct control of protein synthesis. Uncontrolled cell division takes place which leads to cancer.

Preservatives are used to prevent microbial contamination and rancidity. Parabens and ester of parabenzoic acid are examples of preservatives because how effective they are against gram-positive bacteria. The compound phenoxyethanol has the ability to protect cosmetic products against gram-negative skins. A mixture of preservatives is used to protect against different bacterial strains, yeasts, and molds. Vitamin E and BHT are considered antioxidants that prevent oxidation of ingredients that are sensitive. It also protects the skin from free-radical damage.

Additives added to make-up include fragrances and preservatives. But they can account for allergic and irritant reactions. Cosmetic chemists decide to add fragrances to make-up for pleasing scent. Fragrances also hide bad odor of some waxes, oils, and some makeup components. Products that are labeled fragrance-free have no fragrance. If they are labeled unscented, they have no noticeable scent but have enough fragrance additives to cover up the smells of other ingredients. Basically, the purpose of preservatives is to kill microbes.

They are another major kind of additive found in makeup. Bacteria and microorganisms reproduce a lot in warm solutions. If we did not have these preservatives, mascara, foundation, and other makeup becomes a culture for harmful microbes.

Chemicals are added to kill microorganisms or stop their growth. Parabens are examples of preservatives in makeup. Compounds such as butylparaben, ethylparaben, and methylparaben are normally not allergic. But be careful about preservatives called quarternium-l5, formaldehyde, and sorbic acid. These preservatives cause many allergic reactions. Another class of chemical preservatives are called antioxidants. They are listed as product labels such as butylated hydroxyanisole (BHA) and butylated hydroxytoluene (BHT). These additives are added to prevent ingredients combining with oxygen. When oxygen is combined, we call this oxidation, and it can ruin the makeup's color and texture.

Most creams and lotions are emulsions. We can think of an emulsion as two fluids that are immiscible. One of the liquids is dispersed as droplets in another. Oil can be dispersed in water. Fat does not float to the top because of emulsifiers. Water can also be dispersed in the oil phase. The nondispersed liquid is considered to be the continuous phase. Common ingredients in lotion include water, glycerin, and stearic acid. Water is one of the essential ingredients. People who buy moisturizing lotion think it has special ingredients for extra moisture. It might contain substances to moisturize the skin. But most moisturizing lotions have more water content or more pure forms of water. Water and glycerin or glycerol seem to be common ingredients. Glycerol is a humectant that allows the skin to obtain moisture from water in the air.

Oil is another ingredient in lotion. Oils in lotion can vary. They can be solids such as shea butter, mango butter, or coconut butter or they can be liquids such as hazelnut, seed oil, or mineral oil. Lanolin can also be found in lotion. It is a greasy substance. It is wax derived from sheep's wool that ends up softening the skin. Acids are also common lotion ingredients. Citric acid is a preservative and extends the shelf life. Stearic acid is used to change consistency. When lotion is made, it could be fluid. Adding more stearic acid makes the substance thicker. Adding solid oils like shea butter causes less stearic acid to be needed. Vitamins are also added in lotion. Vitamin E benefits the skin by healing of wounds and elasticity. Vitamin C is also included in lotion recipes. It is added for antioxidant properties. It is used to help renew the skin and lessen signs of aging. Fragrance is also added to lotion for those who do not have sensitive skin. The scent of a lotion is what helps the lotion to sell. Those who have sensitive skin should use fragrance-free lotion.

Let us talk about emulsiers. A lot of the emulsifiers are considered surfactants or surface-active agents. They reduce the surface tension of water. The hydrophile-lipophile or HLB balance determines whether the emulsifier surface is active or not. HLB can be determined by the size of the hydrophilic portion and the size of the lipophilic portion. The polarity of the material is important for the HLB system. Polar materials are towards the top of the scale, and nonpolar materials are towards the bottom of the scale. Emulsifier's polar groups orient towards the aqueous phase. The nonpolar groups orient towards the oil phase for the formation of micelles. Structures give stability to hydrogen bonding and weak electrical forces.

Skin-care emulsifiers are divided into groups of two based on ionic charge. Those that dissociate into charged species are ionic. Those materials that do not dissociate are called nonionic. Ionic emulsifiers is classified based on charge. Anionic molecules have negative charges when it is solvated. Fatty acids that react with alkali metals form soaps. The formation of soap is considered to be saponification. If the molecule overall is negative, it can be classified as anionic. Emulsifiers that are positively charged are called cationic. Amphoteric compounds have both negative and positive charges.

Nonionic emulsifiers are better to use for skin-care emulsion due to safety. They are normally grouped together based on similar chemistries. Fatty acids that are present in fats and oils are grouped together based on the length of the carbon chain. Fatty acids are one of the main components of emulsifiers because of their miscibility in both natural and synthetic oils. Polyethylene glycol and ethylene glycol are considered to be PEG esters. The solubility of a PEG ester is based on the number of PEG molecules that has been reacted per molecule of acid. Increasing the number of polar PEG molecules per acid increases the water solubility and the HLB is increased.

Most emollients are considered to be fats and oils which we call lipids. The best emollients have spreading properties, low toxicity, low skin irritation, and the ability to have oxidative stability. Double bonds in some molecules give poor oxidative stability. Saturated fats and oils have no double bonds. There are also unsaturated oils that have double bonds which can react with oxygen when it is heated. Oxidation processes give unpleasant colors and odors in lipids making them rancid and not usable. More likely we will find petroleum-based emollients in formulations since they don't contain double bonds or reactive functional groups. Cyclomethicone and dimethicone are added to increase emolliency.

Essential fatty acids or EFAs present in oils have the ability to replenish lipids that are within skin layers. Fatty alcohols are best used as emollients and emulsion stabilizers. The polar hydroxyl groups orients itself towards the aqueous phase while the fatty side-chains orients itself towards the oil phase. Fatty acids and esters of fatty alcohols are good to use as emollients since they have stability. Polar hydroxyl groups of sterols and alcohols make the grease absorb and hold water. Our skin is made up primarily of water. A lot of oils and emollients are used to take care and protect it. It has low reactivity and good composition.

Moisturizers and emollients differ in their ability of being soluble in water. We need moisture to take care of our healthy skin. Moisturizers that are mainly polar are hygroscopic. In other words, they hold onto water. Measuring transepidermal water loss or TEWL can assess how effective moisturizers are. By applying moisturizer to the skin, the level of moisture is recorded. Eventually, the level of moisture reduces to the tendency of the skin so moisture is released over time. Ingredients that have a high level of moisture in the upper layers of our skin reduce the rate in which water can be lost. Glycerin helps reduce TEWL. Sorbital and sugars are used to hydrate the skin. Aloe has a mixture of polysaccharides, carbohydrates, and minerals. Together, they make a good moisturizer.

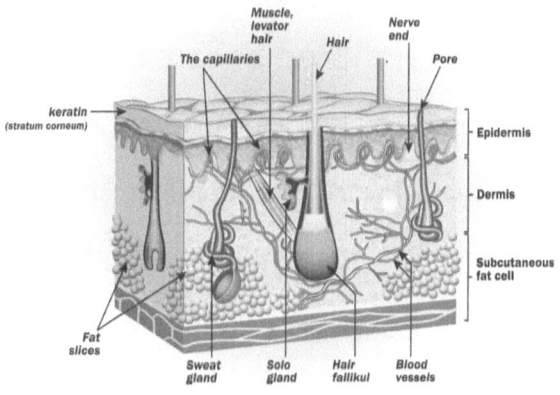

Four skin types include normal skin, dry skin, oily skin, and combination skin. Normal skin has a smooth surface due to oil and moisture content. It is not greasy, and it is not dry. There are also small and barely seen pores. The skin looks clear, and it does not develop spots and blemishes. Little and gentle treatment is needed for people with normal skin. Taking care of the face is always required. Dry skin is different from normal skin. Dry skin has a tendency to flake easily. It is susceptible to wrinkles and lines because it does not retain moisture. Not enough production of sebum by sebaceous glands is produced. Cold weather becomes even more of a problem. Dry skin becomes oily even more. Moisturizer needs to be put on during the day. Moisture-rich cream needs to be put on during the night. Do not overexfoliate since the skin can dry out even further. Exfoliants like sugar, rice bran, or mild acids are the best to use, but they should only be used once a week. You want to make sure you avoid irritation and dryness.

Oily skin can be moderately greasy. This has to do with sebum being over secreted. A lot of oil on the surface of the skin creates dust and dirt from our environment to stick to the oil. Oily skin usually gives rise to blackheads, whiteheads, ugly spots, and pimples. Oily skin has to be cleaned every day. This applies especially in hot or humid weather. It is best to use a moisturizer that is both oil-free and water-based, and it is also a noncomedogenic moisturizer. It is important to carry out exfoliation. Over-exfoliation causes irritation and increases the production of oil. It is best to use exfoliants that have fruit acids. Fine-grained exfoliants could help clear blocked pores.

Combination skin is also common. It consists of both oily and dry skins in different areas. Oily parts are normally found towards a central panel called the T-zone that consists of the forehead, nose, and chin. Dry areas make up the cheeks and areas around the eyes and mouth. Different parts of the face should be treated based on the type of skin. The skin is delicate, and it is more susceptible to irritation, redness, burning, flaking, rashes, and lumpiness. Chemicals, dyes, and fragrances cause irritation. Others include soaps, spice oils, flower oils, spray tans, tanning lotions, shaving creams, temperature changes, excessive exfoliating, threading, waxing, and bleaching. Avoid fragrances, chemical dyes, and those cosmetics that cause skin irritation. Skin type could either be dry, oily, normal, or a combination.

Applying a cosmetic cold cream on the skin, for example, gives a cooling sensation because of evaporation of the alcohol. Skin products include ethanol. Alcohol helps the ability of the components inside the cold cream to dissolve. Having alcohol in the mixture helps putting the cream on the skin, gives a perfume odor, and it also gives a cooling effect on the skin. Evaporation of an alcohol gives a cooling effect because evaporation is an endothermic process or in other words it requires heat. The skin gives the proper amount of heat that is needed to evaporate the alcohol. This leads to a cooling sensation. The alcohol with a hydroxyl group attached to carbon is considered to be a volatile species. Alcohols such as ethanol have low boiling points and high vapor pressures that help with evaporation and which gives a cooling sensation. A higher vapor pressure for a liquid at a specific temperature causes a higher tendency for the molecules to escape to the gas phase.

There are six ways we can take care of our skin. The first one is cleansing. Using a cleanser is the first step. Cleansers can be put on wet skin such as the face and neck. Make sure you avoid the eyes and lips. Cleansing the face once every twenty-four hours should be sufficient. If makeup has been worn to remove extra dirt or oil, then a mild cleanser should be used. If you have oily skin, then you should clean it at least twice per day. Cleansers that are water-based are the best to use. But if you have acne, it is better to use medicated cleansers that contain benzoyl peroxide or salicylic acid. Soap should be avoided for dry and sensitive skin. Soaps are prepared from fats such as coconut oil. Perfumes are added to give the soap a pleasant smell. Soap is considered to be a salt of a long-chain fatty acid. Both ends of a soap have different polarities. The long chain end is both nonpolar and hydrophobic which means "water-fearing". The hydrophobic portion is soluble in nonpolar substances like oil or grease, but they are not soluble in water. The carboxylate salt end is considered to be ionic. It is referred to as hydrophilic which means "water-loving". It is soluble in water but not in oils or grease. Soap is used to clean grease or oil. The nonpolar ends of the soap molecules dissolve in nonpolar fats and oils along with dirt. The polar ends of the soap molecules dissolve in water. Soap molecules coat the oil or grease and form clusters called micelles. Ionic portions of the soap molecules give polarity to micelles and makes them soluble in water. Small globules of oil and fat become coated with soap molecules. They are pulled into the water and are washed away. We need to be careful using soaps since the carboxylate end reacts with cations such as Ca^{2+} and Mg^{2+} that form insoluble substances. Cleansers that are oil-based are good at removing dirt and makeup. It is always good to cleanse the face before putting makeup on.

Masks are a second way to take care of our faces. Facemasks are put on the skin for a certain amount of time, and then the mask gets removed. It is put on a cleanse face making sure to avoid the eyes and lips. Clay-based masks make use of kaolin clay to put oils and chemicals on the skin. It is left on until it is completely dry. The clay then dries absorbing a lot of oil and dirt from the skin and helps clear blocked pores. Clay based masks should only be put on oily skin. Peel masks contain different types of acids or exfoliating agents that exfoliate the skin and other ingredients to hydrate the skin. These masks are left on to dry and then they peel off. If you have dry skin, then you should not use it. Sheet masks, however, are different. They contain a thin cotton or fiber sheet where there are holes cut out for the eyes and lips. Serums and skin treatments are then buried in a thin layer. Sheets can also be soaked for treatment.

Exfoliants is a third way to cleanse the face. They slough off both dry and dead skin. Acids or other chemicals is used to loosen old skin cells. Abrasive substances can also be used to scrub them off. The process of exfoliation evens out rough skin. This helps improve circulation to the skin, clear up blocked pores, and head scars. Exfoliants should be put on wet cleansed skin making sure to avoid the eye area. Abrasive exfoliants or scrubs can be used to rub into the skin by circular motion for around thirty seconds or more. If you have spots with severe flaking, dry skin should be exfoliated in those areas. This should be done only once per week. Some oily skins can tolerate twice weekly use of exfoliation. If you have sore, dry, irritated skin, or lots of dryness or oiliness, then this is caused by over-exfoliation.

Glycolic acid, lactic acid, salicylic acid, malic acid, acetic acid, and citric acid are considered to be chemical exfoliants. They could be in the form of liquids or gels. Some of them might contain abrasives to remove old skin cells. Microfiber brushes can be used to exfoliate the skin. You have to rub them on your face in circular motion.

Creams, lotions, or gels might contain acid to help loosen dead skin cells. Abrasives such as beads or rice bran can be used to scrub dead cells off of the skin.

The fourth way we can take care of our face is through toning. Toners can be used after cleaning the skin and remove any traces of cleanser or makeup in order to maintain the skin's natural pH. Cotton pads can be wiped over the skin. It can also be sprayed on the skin from a spray bottle. Toners normally contain alcohol, water, and herbal extracts of other kinds of chemicals. Toners that have alcohol should be used for oily skins. If you have dry or normal skin, toners that are alcohol-free should be used.

Moisturizing is a fifth way to clean the face. Moisturizers are considered to be creams or lotions that hydrate the skin and help retain moisture. Some of them have oils, herbal extracts, or chemicals to help with controlling the oil or reducing irritation. NightGels, creams, and lotions are abrasive exfoliants. It can be applied to creams and, they are better hydrating than dry creams. Some moisturizers are tinted and contain a small amount of foundation. This provides light coverage for minor blemishes and to even out skin tones. Avoid putting moisturizers near the lips and around the eyes.

Regardless of the type of skin, it needs to be moisturized and protected (spf). Using a moisturizer reduces flaking and dryness. It could also help prevent wrinkles from forming. If you have dry skin, it is best to use oil-based moisturizers with ingredients so the skin can retain moisture and protect it from dryness, heat, or cold. If you have normal skin, you have many moisturizers to choose from. Light lotions or gels are the best ones to use. Moisturizers that are water-based should be put on oily skin. Moisturizers that are medicated and that also have tea extracts or fruit enzymes control oil production and could also treat acne. Our skin around the eyes is thin and sensitive. Eye creams are considered to be light lotions or gels. Some contain ingredients like caffeine or Vitamin K that are used in order to reduce puffiness and dark circles seen under the eye.

The sixth and last way to protect our face is to avoid the sun as much as possible. The hot rays of the sun can cause a lot of damage to the skin including sunburns and skin cancer. The sun also exposes us to UVA and UVB radiation that causes uneven skin tone and dries out the skin. This reduces elasticity and encourages the formation of wrinkles. We should use sunscreen to protect ourselves from the skin. It also won't hurt to check the daily newspaper for the ultraviolet ratings index for the day. It gives a scale from 1 to 10 where 1 is the lowest amount and 10 is the highest amount of exposure of ultraviolet rays from the sun for the day.

Any skin that will be exposed to sunlight, sunscreen should be put on. Sunscreens can be in the form of creams, gels, or lotions. The SPF number indicates how effective it is to protect the skin from the radiation of the sun. If you have oily skin, it is best to choose non-comodegenic sunscreens. If you have dry skin, it is best to choose sunscreens with moisturizers that help keep the skin hydrated. If you have sensitive skin, choose hypoallergenic sunscreen that is not scented. It might be a good idea to put it on a small spot to check to see if it does not irritate the skin.

It is important to get into the habit by carefully reading labels of ingredients and descriptions. Prone skin is a challenge facing several people. The best thing to do is to pick products labeled noncomedogenic. This means that they don't promote whitehead or blackhead pimples. You should also choose products that are nonacnegenic. This means they don't form any kind of pimple. It is also best to select products that are labeled oilfree. But do check the product if it contains greasy substances like lanolin, petrolatum, or emollient esters. Foundations do their best to prevent acne breakouts with ingredients such as salicylic acid. Salicylic acid fights microbes. Benzoyl peroxide acts as a drying agent. These ingredients dry the skin. But keep in mind a large number of people (10% of the population) are allergic to benzoyl peroxide.

Dry skin can also be a problem. Dry skin becomes a problem for older women. Ingredients you should avoid include alcohols such as ethanol, methanol, and other types of alcohols. These dry the skin. It is a good idea not to use foundations or cover sticks that have powder in them. Some products have good drying agents. Cetearyl and stearyl are considered to be fatty alcohols. They help moisturize dry skin. Other good quality ingredients include lactic acid, glycolic acid, and urea. These nonoily compounds are called humectants, and they do not add moisture to the skin. Humectants cover the skin with a protective film that prevents water in the skin from evaporating. Sensitive skin and allergic reactions affect people of all ages. If the product is labeled "hypoallergenic" (a made up marketing term by Este Lauder in the 1960s), then they are less likely to cause allergies than regular products. Products that are labeled hypoallergenic normally do not contain fragrances, preservatives, and other causes of irritation and allergic reactions. Keep in mind these products are not 100% allergy proof. Some of the ingredients can cause allergic reactions.

Although products labeled allergy tested, sensitivity tested, and dermatologist tested are on makeup labels, they do not tell us exactly whether the product passed the test or not and if it was done in an independent laboratory. If you are prone to allergies or have sensitive skin, it might be a good idea to test the new makeup on a different part of the body such as on your arm for a few weeks before applying the makeup on your face. If you wear contact lens you should be careful using mascara, eye shadow, and other eye makeup. Avoid mascara that has silk or nylon fibers and water-based mascara that falls into the eye. Frosted eye shadow is also not a good idea because the iridescent particles can fall into your eye and stick to the contact lens. It is possible this can scratch the eye's own lens which is in the cornea. You also need to reduce bacterial infection and contaminating particles. Be sure to wash your hands and put in your contacts before applying makeup. There are three basic safety warnings we should consider. The first safety warning is never put on mascara while in the car or when the vehicle is moving. A common injury when putting up makeup is scratching the eye using a mascara wand. The scratch itself is not the health hazard. It is the sight infection that can be threatening if the scratch is not treated right away. The second safety warning to consider is to never put makeup on that is spoiled. If the product does not look consistent, has a foul odor, or if there is a change in color, then it is possible it could have microbes. These can cause infections. Don't add water or saliva to the makeup that is dried. This will only add more contamination with microbes, and it can cause microbes with the liquid to be harmful. When you are not using makeup, it should be tightly closed and away from sunlight. Sunlight destroys preservatives. The third safety warning to consider is to never share makeup. Sharing makeup passes microbes back and forth. This is also a problem with sharing of testers at cosmetic counters. Counter makeup samples can be contaminated with bacteria, mold, and/or microbes. It is a good idea to test lipstick on your hand. Be sure to ask for a new cotton swab to test other makeup products.

It is important to understand emulsion chemistry and skin physiology when making personal care products. The difference between over the counter products and professional products is that professional products have been carefully researched in laboratories. You are taking more of a risk using over the counter products. A lot of work has to be done to take care of us. Choosing the right makeup product for our faces is crucial if we are going to achieve the best results of our facial appearance. A lot of the cosmetics discussed including primers, lipstick, concealers, foundation, face powder, blush, bronzer, and mascara needs to be carefully applied on the woman's face. Understanding the chemistry of each of these cosmetics can help make important decisions. It is good know something about the color, the bases used, bulking agents, waxes, thickeners, active ingredients, emulsions, moisturizers, sunscreens, preservatives, surfactants, and emollients. These determine the outcome of the product that is being used for the female. Taking care of the skin is just as important when choosing the appropriate cosmetic. Different skin types and the right use of facial care can help us look younger, natural, and appear nice in public. Despite all of the benefits looking nice using cosmetics, it is also important to consider safety features. Understanding healthy uses of cosmetics versus toxicity can keep us from making mistakes by choosing the wrong products. Taking care of our skin is important for our health. The following pictures show chemical formulas of food and cosmetic preservatives.

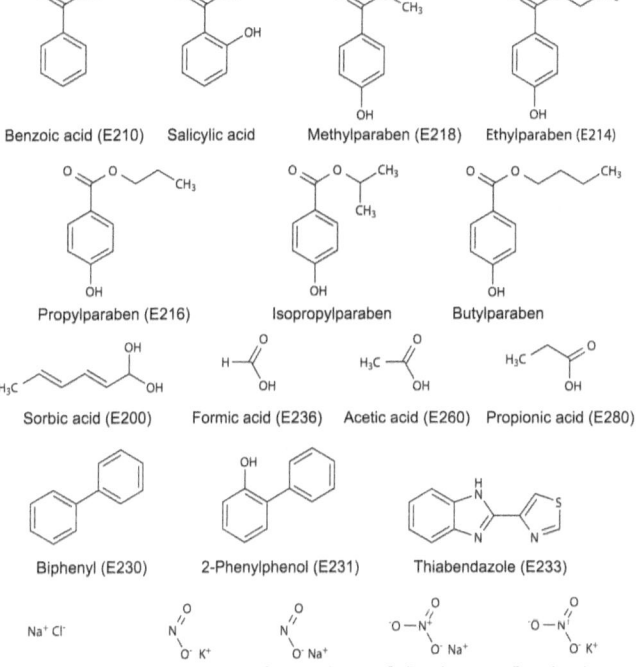

Benzoic acid (E210) Salicylic acid Methylparaben (E218) Ethylparaben (E214)

Propylparaben (E216) Isopropylparaben Butylparaben

Sorbic acid (E200) Formic acid (E236) Acetic acid (E260) Propionic acid (E280)

Biphenyl (E230) 2-Phenylphenol (E231) Thiabendazole (E233)

Sodium chloride Potassium nitrite (E249) Sodium nitrite (E250) Sodium nitrate (E251) Potassium nitrate (E252)

Chapter 4

Cosmetics I

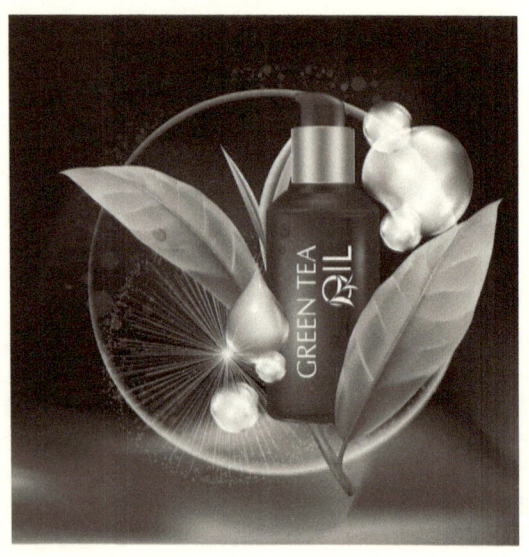

Countering and highlighting are excellent methods for enhacing facial features. But it has to be done correctly. Contouring involves using shadows to slim the face and minimize features that are undesirable.

Highlighting is using light to bring foward features of the face. Strobing is another trend going on in makeup. Strobing has to do with layering highlighters on high points on the face with different degrees of reflecting ability to define features on the face. Extreme contouring is also becoming popular.

Keep in mind not all products are going to work on everyone. Reading labels and learning the truth about mineral makeup and palm oils is important. A lot of people are concerned about what they put on their skin. We do our best to eat healthy and exercise whether it is at a gym or somewhere else of our liking. We do our best to make sure the skin does not absorb cancer-causing chemicals whether we put it on our faces or any other part of our body.

It is not good to trust any labels on products. If something is labelled natural, then that does not mean it is from pure nature. A bottle labeled organic probably contains 5-15%, but it could contain unhealthy ingredients. Natural skin care is important for our bodies. One of the best facial moisturizers is a dry cream. It is used on the face to moisturize and protect the face. A good body wash are Magic Pure Castile classic soaps. They are biodegradable and vegetable-based. Typical fragrances include Almond, Peppermint, Citrus, Rose, and Lavender.

Eye Cream with organics are a lot more healthier. Cleansing gels are also excellent. These are recently bought by a cosmetic/pharmaceutical company. These natural and nondrying cleansing gels clean the skin and pores from impurities. It does not cause excessive dryness. Microfoliants are also excellent cosmetics. It is probably not a good idea to exfoliate on a daily basis. Exfoliate a couple of times a week makes it better to slough off dead skin cells. It contains a rice-based enzyme powder. It also gets rid of debris. It also unclogs pores, and it has no artificial fragrance or color.

Emollient body lotions has sunscreen and moisturizing properties and which has no parabens. Body shea butter is a moisture cream. It contains the antioxidants Vitamans A and E as well as arnica extract and sodium hyaluronate which is an oil-free mixture. Let us also not forget that natural crystal deodorants are good to use since they do not have aluminum.

Jojoba Oil works for very dry skin. It is both gentle and natural and works as a good makeup remover. Coconut cream contain the ingredients coconut oil, aloe vera, and distilled lanolin. Organic purifying facial cleanser is a facial cleanser that also works very good. Coconut Oil is excellent to moisturize skin, use it for dry air, and apply it as a foundation primer to remove makeup. It is one of the best organic beauty products. It is not good to put unhealthy ingredients that could get absorbed in our bloodstream. You can use coconut oil as a body moisturizer, exfoliating the face, use as a great hair conditioner, use to treat acne and heal wounds, use to remove makeup, use as a foundation primer, use to fight dandruff, and use as a body scrub.

Mineral makeup is also good to stay healthy. Unlike other kinds of makeup, most mineral makeup does not have preservatives, mineral oil, parabens, chemical dyes, and (synthetic) fragrances. Fillers are inert ingredients used to give bulk, lubricity, and texture to the product. It helps promote healing and reduces irritation. Binders and petrochemicals are just as important. Women with sensitive skin can easily breakout. Makeup that comes in powdered form such as eyeshadows, foundations, blush, bronzers that uses 100% mineral makeup is the best choice. Bismuth oxychloride is also used in cosmetics. People have the ability to inhale or ingest bismuth. It can also be absorbed through the skin. Some people feel bismuth is nontoxic in small amounts; however, enough exposure of this element can produce headache, diarrhea, nausea, and pain.

Using staples in the kitchen is also a good way to take care of the skin. You can save time and money rather than purchasing expensive products. Using homemade versions of brown sugar body, oatmeal scrubs face, lip scrub which one can use honey and brown sugar, making our own baby wipes, milk bath recipes, sugar wax recipes, organic extra virgin coconut oil used as an overall body product to lock in your own moisturizer, using apple cider vinegar that helps add shine to limp locks, olive oil as eye makeup remover, making hair conditioner, making face masks from simple ingredients, making tinted lip balm, organic extra virgin coconut oil as foundation primer, using lemon as a toner, and highlight hair with chamomile tea can all be used to take care of the skin rather than purchase expensive products. Regardless of what products you decide to purchase it is always good to know databases whenever shopping for products. EWG's Skin Deep Cosmetics Database can be used to carry out research on the best and healthy cosmetics. Their website address is http://www.ewg.org/skindeep/

It is also good to look for sulfate-free shampoos. There are some sulfates found in shampoos and facial cleansers that causes it to lather. It is probably best to avoid shampoos/face wash with foaming agents such as sodium laureth sulfate and ammonium laureth sulfate. Products that end with "eth" have the ability to test positive for 1,4-dioxane. The chemical 1,4-dioxane is a clear and colorless organic compound that is a liquid at room temperature. It is known as a human carcinogen. Examples of products that end with "eth" are sodium laureth sulfate, oleth, myreth, polyethylene glycol, and ceteareth. Avoid the following mistakes when shampooing your hair. It is best to deep condition curly hair. Some people don't wet their hair thoroghly, use too much or too little shampoo, don't pay attention to the scalp, don't rinse and repeat, don't thoroughly rinse the shampoo out of the hair, skip the conditioner and not apply it thoroughly, don't comb the hair in the shower, the conditioner is not thoroghly rinsed out of the hair, and they don't finish the hair with a cold water rinse. These are mistakes when people don't shampoo their hair.

The best moisturizers are oils. Keep it simple when it comes to moisturizing and stick to oils. Extra virgin coconut oils, almond oil, olive oil, and jojoba oil work really good to hydrate the skin for both the face and the body. It is also a good idea to safely color your hair. It is best to use organic vegetable-base dye. As for soaps, use them in the shower and use cleansers for the face. It has been known that soaps strip the skin for its moisture. It is best to stick to natural soaps made of moisturizing ingredients which include goat milk, shea butter, clear glyercin, olive oil, or liquid castile. When taking a shower, using castille soaps are good to use because they are biodegradable and vegetable-based. Jojoba wax comes from Jojoba. It is used in candles, soaps, and castles.

There are some people who have dry skin, oily skin, or eczema. Go for the basic cleanser possible. Dermalogica has a reputation for making excellent facial cleansers. Other people use cleaning cream. Some people may use organic milk used as a cleaner. It is also possible to mix honey with milk if there is dry skin. Salt can be mixed with warmed milk if there is dry skin. However, it may or may not work on all people.

Hair masks and rinses can be used to save money. Basic ingredients can be found in most kitchens. Fine hair can be oil and susceptible to product build up. Spray hair with a vinegar rinse to get rid of product build-up. You can even add to the body with sea salt sprays. If you have blonde fair chlorine can turn it green. In fact, chlorine is harmful to the hair. It dries out and ruins natural color. There is no need to buy a shampoo product for swimmers. All that is needed is an apple vinegar rinse. Dandruff can also be treated naturally. Use flaxseed then follow it with apple cider vinegar. This is great for fighting yeast and bacteria. You can even make hair conditioners by using basic ingredients such as extra virgin olive oil, brown sugar, and an essential oil. Baking soda shampoo followed with vinegar spritz is better than commercial shampoos. Why buy shaving cream. Olive oil or hair conditioner can be used to shave the legs since it is moisturizing. Wax also works since it is natural, lasts longer, and has better results.

It may also be a good idea to skip the makeup remover. Use either almond oil or olive oil with a cotton pad and warm water. People with dry and/or curly hair end up using Moroccanoil hair products. These products have argan oil. They come from a rich source of Vitamin E and essential fatty acids. It can be applied to the hair and skin. Argan oil is considered to be organic. Moroccanoil brands contain other ingredients such as silicones that are not organic. They still do their best to control frizz.

It may also not be a bad idea to avoid palm oils. Exposure of the sun with palm oils has caused wrinkles and could cause skin cancer. But don't avoid the sun. Sunshine compels the body to make Vitamin D. Vitamin D is important to have because it strengthens immunity and bones. It also heals acne, rashes, psoriasis, and eczema. It is probably better to expose your skin during the early and late hours instead during the brightest times during the day. Some people supplement using Vitamin D pills, but it is always a good idea to check with your doctor. It is usually the hottest between 11 am to 3 pm. Getting the sun's benefits on your skin is when the sun's rays are not at the brightest point. During the sun's strongest hours, put on sunscreen and wear a hat. Some people who hang out at the beach or pool decide to stay under an umbrella or during the shade.

If you want to have a gorgeous tan, then build it up. It is best to know more about the health of your skin. Ultraviolet exposure of rays from the sun gives premature aging and cancer. Avoid a sunburn by using a 20 SPF sunscreen. Spending about 20 minutes in the sun will help build up your tan. You might end up having a great tan without a burn. It is a good idea to put sunscreen at least 20 minutes before exposing yourself to the sun. Sunscreen needs time to allow it to soak in. Once the sunscreen is absorbed, put on your bathing suit and cover-up. Completely cover just about every inch of the skin with sunscreen. If you spend more than 2 hours outside, reapply the sunscreen which ends up seating off and losing its resiliency. If you are swimming it is good to reapply it every time you sit down.

Suncreen screens the skin to get the amounts of daily Vitamin D. It is probably better to use sunscreen on the face to make sure you don't get wrinkles. Only skip putting sunscreen on the legs and arms during the day unless you decide to be outside and your skin burns quickly. You should be able to know how much Vitamin D is needed by exposing your skin to the sun without being burned. Perhaps it may be best to go without sunscreen during the mornings and afternoons, but wear it from 11 am - 3 pm. Perhaps during the winter, only wear sunscreen on the face and allow both the hands and arms get some sun. It is also a good idea to choose sunscreens. Go for at least 30 SPF or a 60 SPF if you have sensitive skin. Make sure the sunscreen you are using includes UVA and UVB protection. When applying sunscreen, slather it everywhere and then do a second-round on sun-susceptible areas. It is best to start with the nose, forehead, and cheeks. Then move to the tips of the ears, back of the neck, chest, shoulders, knees, and back of the legs. If you ever feel your skin gets hot, find a shade.

Deodorant is another cosmetic that should be applied carefully. Some people have a concern about putting aluminum or other chemicals under their arms. Using natural deodorants is best. Some popular items include a deodorant that does not have aluminum. The trick is to apply the stone to a large swath under the arm and not where the hair grows. You might need to wet the stone twice. It is also good to leave the top off the cap so the stone to dry before closing it. Using these two kinds of deodorants avoids yellow staining that normally comes with aluminum deodorants.

Let us take a look at antiperspirants. Antiperspirants clog up pores so wetness does not leak out. Aluminum chloride clogs up pores. Aluminum chloride is not good because it is linked to Alzheimer's disease and also to breast cancer. A lot of doctors warn people to avoid using aluminum in beauty products. Some people also like to avoid using parabens. Making a facial scrub or finding a good facial scrub to buy would be a wise decision. It is probably not a good idea to exfoliate daily. Exfoliating a couple times a week to slough off dead skin cells should do the job. The skin should look amazing after using it one time with a good exfoliant. Making scrubs using brown sugar on the face or just simply use a microfoliant. Making your own body scrubs using basic ingredients such as salt or sugar, body oil, and a warm bath can also save you money. Treating dandruff naturally is also a good idea. Using homemade dandruff remedies is better for the hair and scalp than using chemicals found in dandruff shampoos. Flax seed oil is one of the main homemade ingredients that can be used to treat dandruff.

Buffers are considered to be solutions that resist changes in pH of acidity and alkanlinity when small amounts of acid or alkali are added. They are chemical compounds that occur naturally in sugar cane, milk, and fruits. Alpha hydroxy acids used in cosmetic products are glycolic acid from sugar cane and lactic acid from sour milk. Other alpha hydroxy acids include citric acid from oranges and lemons. There are even products in the market used to exfoliate and cleanse the skin. They do their best to reduce skin wrinkling, even out skin tones, and smooth the skin. They are put on the surface of the skin which removes dead surface cells and improve the skin's appearance. Alpha hydroxy acids are also used as pH adjusters. They make sure products are not too acidic or basic. They are also mild and nonirritating. Apples and other fruits contain carboxylic acids and function as pH adjusters and are used in mild exfoliation in cosmetic formulations.

Organic Buffer Systems. First Set

Compounds such as triethanolamine, diethanolamine, and ethanolamine are clear viscous liquids that have odors like ammonia. Triethanolamine is used in cosmetics and personal care products such as eyeliners, eye shadows, mascara, blushes, fragrances, hair dyes, sunscreens, wave sets, skin cleansing products, and make-up bases and foundations. Triethanolamine, diethanolamine, and ethanolamine form emulsions and reduce surface tension of substances to be emulsified so water-soluble and oil-solube ingredients mix well together. They even control the pH of cosmetics and other personal care products.

Triethanolamine, malic acid, sodium phosphate, calcium carbonate, alpha hydroxy acid, disodium phosphate, and trisodium phosphate are considered to be white crystalline solids. Sodium phosphate ingredients are found in the formulation of bath products, mouthwashes, colognes, hair dyes, skin care products and makeup. Both sodium phosphate and disodium phosphate are used as buffering agents and are used as corrosion inhibitors. Trisodium phosphate is used as a pH adjuster. The compounds sodium phosphate, calcium carbonate, and zinc carbonate are salts from carbonic acid. These ingredients are white powders. The carbonate salts are found in bath products, makeup products oral care products, skin, hair, and personal products.

The compounds calcium carbonate is used as a buffering agent. Both magnesium carbonate and potassium carbonate are used as pH adjusters. Malic acid is a dicarboxylic acid that contributes to the taste of apples. Both malic acid and sodium malate are used in a wide variety of cosmetics and personal care products. They even control the pH of cosmetic products.

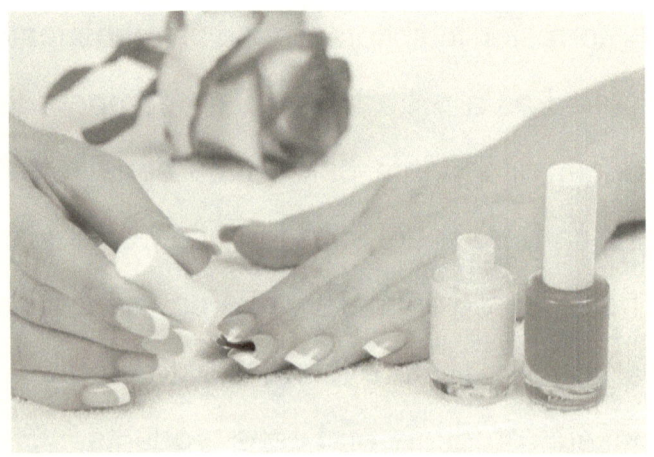

Nail polish also seems to be popular among women. It originated in China. Nail polish is also called nail varnish. It is considered to be a laquer that is applied to human fingernails and toenails. It is also used to decorate and protect nail plates. Many processes that make nail polish have been enhanced for decoration and used to make sure there is no cracking of the fingernails. Nail polish consists of a solution containing an organic polymer and other compounds. Nail polish is made of a film-foaming polymer dissolved in a volatile organic solvent. Nitrocellulose is dissolved in either butyl acetate or ethyl acetate. This is considered to be a basic formulation. Plasticizers such as dibutylphthalate and camphor can be added to give non-brittle films. Dyes and pigments can also be added. Examples include chromium oxide greens, stannic oxide, chromium hydroxide, iron oxide, ferric ferrocyanide, carmine, titanium oxide, manganese violet, and ultramarine. Opalescent pigment which adds glitter can also be added. The color comes from mica, bismuth, oxychloride, natural pearls, and even aluminum powder.

Polymers that are adhesive makes sure the nitrocellulose stays on the nail's surface. A modifier that can be used is tosylamide-formaldehyde resin. Thickening agents can also be added to keep the particles sparkling while it is sealed inside the bottle. An example of a thickener is stearalkonium hectorite. Thickening agents have the property called thixotropy. The solutions can be viscous when they are still, but they can still flow freely when they are agitated. Both of these properties enable the mixture to give the film that solidifies. Ultraviolet stabilizers can also be added. They resist color changes when the film is dried and exposed to light. An example of a stabilizer is benzophenone-1. Storing nail polish in a refrigerator extends its shelf life.

Choosing nail polish is always a concern. It might be best to skip drugstore brands. Caring about natural skincare is important in order to live long. Consider "3-free" and "5-free" polishes. These polishes don't contain awful ingredients found in drugstores. Nails are actually porous. Some of the cheap brands on nail polishes contain toxins. Using formaldehyde over a long period of time causes cancer. Dibutyl phthalate is not good for the reproductive system. Toluene is harmful to unborn fetuses.

Some nail polish brands are 3-free and 5-free. They don't have toxic ingredients. 5-free polishes exclude camphor and formaldehyde resin in the products. Both of these have been known to be allergens.

Formaldehyde is awful. Even though it is a nail hardener, it has the ability to contact dermatitis for those with allergies. Inhaling camphor in large doses causes problems too. These ingredients can be hazardous for those people who pain their fingers and toes often. Nail polish can be removed either by nail pads or nail polish remover. The remover consists of an organic solvent and may include oils, scents, and coloring. The most common solvent is acetone. Acetone is powerful enough to remove artificial nails which are made up of acrylic and gel nails. Ethyl acetate is also an active ingredient in nonacetone nail polish removers which also has isopropyl alcohol. Ethyl acetate is normally the solvent in nail polish. Keep in mind there are some scary ingredients in nail polish. Formaldehyde is a carcinogen, and it is connected to lung cancer and nasal cancer. Dibutyl phthalate or DBP is linked to reproductive issues, and toluene affects the nervous system. It can cause dizziness, headaches, eye irritation, nausea, birth defects, liver and kidney damage, and developmental abnormalities.

Let us take a look at lip liners. Some of them are waterproof and have major ingredients include Vitamin E, cottonseed oil, and jojoba oil. Lips stay hydrated and smooth. Some have one side highlight lips. The other side helps filll them in. Both sides work together to give you the best shape. If you are using the shape side of the pencil, use it to highlight the cupid's bow and outline the lips for a full and better look. Apply the definer on the inside, follow the same outline, and then blend it with lip brush.

Some products have an intense waterproof formula. It has a precise glide-on application. Fill in the lip and apply liptick on top. Use it to line and define. Some products have stay on lip contouring pencil works best for those who don't want to spend a lot of money. It has wooden pencil sharpeners. It is nontransferable long wear liner, and it protects against lipstick both bleeding and feathering. Some products have a liner retractable pencil does not need to be sharpened. The Semi-matte finish stays on lips. It is used as a semi-matte lip color or you can line it with lip stick. It is important to get the most out of your lipstick. Wear it as a lipstain. Wear it as a tinted lip balm. Turn it matte. Wear it as a cream blush. Liquid lipsticks with ultimate staying power.

Lip Balm is another excellent product to use. It is available in different shades such as lighter and darker colors of neutrals, pinks, and red. It is 100% natural, and it does not get disgusting in the corners of the mouth like some of the other lip balms. However, there is no sun protection. You will need a base coat of lip balm that has a SPF 15 or higher. You will need to keep reapplying the product sometimes throughout the day. The balm will feel soft and creamy. There should be a soothing relief of dryness.

If you choose to vary the color from tinted lip balms, it would be best to try a base coat that has different types of balms. Using a harder balm underneath gives a lighter color on top. A softer balm or petroleum jelly gives a glossier finish. Apply the tinted balm to the lips that will give you the most color. Do this to your lips more than two times. Make the base coat a sun-protective balm so you can avoid wrinkles and skin cancer. Dark color can be intense to look with SPF that is underneath.

Some women out there would like to make their lip appear more fuller. Adding lip gloss is a good technique. They give the illusion you have plump lips. Glossy lipsticks seem to work better than matte lipsticks. It is also a good idea to use a lip liner to line the lips outside the natural lip line. Put liner outside the natural lip line and then put a bit of gloss in the middle of the bottom lip and then put the lips together. Also use makeup to plump up lips. Do note that lip plumpers do work. However, the effect is temporary. Some of the formulas contain a lip-plumping ingredient like MaxLip. It stimulates collagen and it has the ability to boos hydration. There are other ingredients that help retain moisture. If you want your lips to last longer, use lip creams that have peptides or collagen boosters.

Let us take a look at some tips on how to apply lipstick. If you wear red lipstick, it is best to keep the rest of the makeup light. If you use heavy makeup for the eyes, then it is best to keep the mouth light with a beautiful gloss or with a light lip color that does not stand out in front of others. If you want to get nude lips which match well with smokey eyes, cover the lips with concealer or foundation before using lip gloss. The lips ends up looking colorless. If you want to plump the lips just apply liner to the outside of the natural lip line. Then put a gloss in the middle of the bottom of the lip and put the lips together.

When choosing a lipstick, it is best to choose one that works for you and not for the one your friend uses. The best lipstick shade should be 2 or darker than the natural lip color. There is no one best method applying lipstick. Some women use a brush, their middle finger, or applying it from the tube itself. Lipstick can last longer if you fill in the lips with the liner first. Use a nude liner when using a light lipstick. Then put the lipstick on top. Lip gloss can wear off fast. However, if you use a liner, then the gloss sticks to it. Applying a long-lasting lip stain can stay on for hours. It is even possible to line before or after applying lipstick or gloss. It is also a good idea to never use a dark liner that has light lipstick. The liner needs to match the lipstick or gloss. If you have a bad shade of lipstick do not throw it away.

Make a really good lip color by blending lipsticks you don't like. Coloring lips with a darker liner before applying a lipstick that can be too bright.

Do your best to keep the lipstick from staining others. It has been researched that the average woman can consume about six pounds of lipstick throughout her lifetime. The ingredients in lipstick should not harm you. They are broken down by stomach acids. If you want to keep lipstick off the teeth, then after you apply the lipstick, use your index finger and put it in your mouth and then pull it out. Any excess lipstick should come off the finger rather than the teeth. Lipstick can be similar to blush, but you should never use blush as a lipstick. If you are going to use lipstick as a blush, then dab a few dots on the apples of the cheeks and blend it well. Having moistured skin will help the lipstick blend better.

As we get older, the lips thin out. Avoid matte and gloss and use a creamy lipstick. Be cautious when using dark lipsticks. If you want to camouflage yellow teeth, use lipstick with a bluish undertone. Shades that work best include violets, wines, pinks, or plums. If you ever break your lipstick, then use a tissue and wave a match under the broken piece of lipstick. When it becomes melted, then put it back on the base and put it inside the refrigerator but leave it uncovered for about a half an hour. If you have a little bit of lipstick inside the tube, scrape the remaining bits with a cotton swab and then mix it with vaseline or a lip gloss in a lipstick palette. It is best to use a lip brush.

There are going to be organic products that are not going to work for everyone. A lot of people seem content using coconut oil, aloe vera, chamomile, and green teas. There are some oils, however, that can exacerbate pimples or acne if your skin is oily. There are some products derived from fruits that sting the skin and they cause rashes or other skin problems. Some people say lemon juice is one of the best natural toner for the skin. But lemons are really acidic and have a low pH. They are too harsh. Knowing what works and what does not work for the skin is important.

Ask yourself is your face shape round, square, long, heart, or oval. You would have to measure your face. Everyone has at least one of six face shapes. These include round, square, oblong, heart, oval, or diamond.

Get a ruler or tape measure and start with the forehead. Measure the forehead at the widest point. Measure the width across your cheekbones. Measure the jawline at the widest point. Measure the length of the face by using the "cross shape method". Use a ruler under the eyes and measure ear to ear. Stop at where the ear begins. Put the ruler at the top of the forehead at the hairline and measure the chin. You should have a ratio of width to length.

The heart-shaped face or the inverted-triangle face is wider at the forhead and then narrow down along the jawline. Side-swept bangs look great on the heart-shaped face. The pointy chin looks like the focal point on the face. Side-swept bangs give attention to the eyes and cheekbones. Brow-grazing fringe do a good job drawing attention to the eyes and away from the chin. Short hair also looks good on heart-shaped faces. Using long hair with long layers graze your cheek bones.

The square face is another type of face shape. If the width of the forehead, cheekbones, and jaw are equal, a sharp and angular feature including sharp jawline, and a cross ratio of 1 to 1/2 or 1 to 1 then your face is considered to be a square face. Women who have strong angular features do a better job aging. Texture in the form of curls or perhaps choppy ends look good on square face. Shags also look good. You can also use super short and edgy cuts. You can even use long and sleek styles with layers starting from the jawline and then continuing downward. Long bobs and side-swept bangs also look great.

The classic round face is also another type of face shape. The width of the jaw, cheekbones, and forhead are all equal. The jaw is a bit rounded instead of angular. Round faces have soft features. The cross ratio is 1 to 1. Round faces are soft and have nonagular features and full cheeks. Those who have round faces makes their faces appear longer and learner. You should be able to create less volume around the face.

Use cuts that fall below the chin such as the long bob hairstyle. Soft graduated layers makes the face appear slimmer and removes bulk and weight from the sides. Wisps does not emphasize the roundness of the face. Use long or side-swept bangs. It is also a good idea to avoid one-length blunt cuts only if you have short hair. It is also a good idea not to use curly short hair.

Grow the curls to shoulder-length or more or better yet flat iron them.

The diamond face is also another type of face shape. Diamond faces are the widest at the cheekbones. The jawline and forehead have the same length but are narrower than the cheeks. Hairstyles on diamond faces look great on square faces shapes too.

The oblong face is another kind of shape. Long face shapes are considered to be longer than them being wide. If the cross shape ratio is 1 to more than 1.5, then your face falls into the face shape zone. The best haircut is the one that does not drag the face down but adds width. Bangs are good to use since they can hid a big forehead. Brow-skimming, side-swept bangs, or blunt bangs work best. When getting haircuts, chin-length bobs are good to have since they create width. The stylist should the cut the hair tiny bit shorter in the back so it looks more attractive. Curls and waves also look good since they add width to the face. Long hair can drag the face down. Long layers can turn out to work with pieces hitting the nose, the chin, and collarbone. A v-shaped style works good where the length is in the back and the sides and front of the hair appear shorter.

The oval face is another kind of shape. You have an oval face if the length of the face equals 1 1/2 times the width of the face. This is the most versatile face shape. Women can wear almost any hairstyle. Angular bobs work best that shows off your chin for beautiful bone structure. Side-swept bangs or blunt work best with great eyes. It is best to avoid short layers which add height on top of the head. Short layers make the face look long. Avoiding a blunt cut if you have thick or curly hair. Don't go for short hair if you have curly hair.

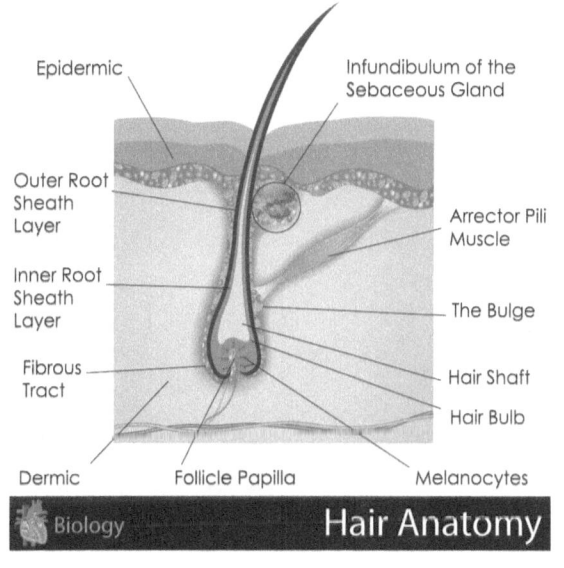

Epidermic

Infundibulum of the Sebaceous Gland

Outer Root Sheath Layer

Arrector Pili Muscle

Inner Root Sheath Layer

The Bulge

Fibrous Tract

Hair Shaft

Hair Bulb

Dermic   Follicle Papilla   Melanocytes

Biology   Hair Anatomy

Chapter 5

Cosmetics II

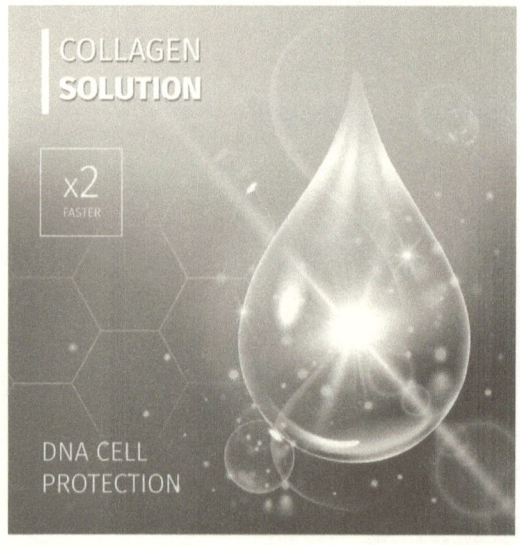

Eyeshadow application requires careful thought. You have to choose the right eyeshadow palette for eye color. Then you need to figure out how to use the various shades on the lid. First you need to prime your lid. Sweep a primer over the lids before applying eyeshadow. You can use your finger or a Q-tip to apply a primer. Next sweep a neutral color over the lids. Choose a neutral shade instead of the darkest and the lightest. Sweep the color over the entire lid up to the crease. A neutral sweep of shadow is considered to be the shadow base to build the rest of the look. A neutral color can make the eyes bigger and cover any lid discoloration. A medium eyeshadow brush is a good tool for eyeshadow application.

The next step is to blend a darker color to your crease. Start from the inside of the eye with a thinner line that grows thicker extending to the outside of the crease. The lids should match and blend. Choose a darker color from a 3-color palette. Choose the third darkest color if you have a 4-color palette. If there is no palette that is being used, it is best to use a color in the same family as a neutral color. Use a brush that is meant for the crease and then apply the crease. The next step is to add highlighter above the crease. If the eyes need more color, then take the lightest color in the palette and blend it above the crease. Keep the color off the browbone. Lighter shades are better. It is best to stay away from the dark shades over here. Blending is important when it comes to eyeshadow. Both of the lids needs to match. The colors should look like a rainbow as if there is a blending from light to a dark to a light color again. The last step would be to put a light shade inside the corner of the eye. If you want to open up the eyes, use your pinkie finger and touch the lightest color of the palette. Then put your pinkie finger inside the corner of the eye. This should make the eyes appear wider and more alive. Just make sure you don't press too much.

When selecting an eye shadow palette, it is best to consider your eye color. The eyes need to pop out. Use a contrasting color palette on the lids. Golds and browns look good on blue eyes. Pinks and browns look good on green eyes. Blues, greens, deep purple, and deep jewel colors look good on brown or dark brown eyes. Nevertheless, it is always good to get professional help when choosing colors. Be cautious when using shimmer eye shadows. Shimmer has the ability to make the eyes pop. It does, however, highlight heavy lids, lines, and wrinkles. Create a "nude" lid and apply a bit of gold shimmer to the browbone. It looks great! Get rid of freebie foam applicators. Brushes are good to use for eyeshadow application. Use a medium-sized brush for the neutral color and another one for the crease. You can also get a smaller blending brush for the highlighter color and an angled brush can be used to apply eyeshadow as a liner. Using eye shadow as eyeliner is important. Use the darkest color in the makeup palette as an eyeliner. Use a small rounded brush, dip it into a dark brown color, and then sweep it under bottom lashes. Go over it with a finger to smudge it. Use an angled brush to get a precise line. Take a brush and dip it in water first to make a liquid liner from the shadow. If you want your shadow to last, it is best to set it with a primer first. Complicated eyeshadow involves a lot of blending. Creating a smokey eye is common for a lot of women. Keep the color to the lid and under the lower lashline. Do not extend the color above the crease.

There is a way to make the eyes look more brighter. Press a little bit of light eyeshadow in the inside corner of the eye. The eyes look brighter and more awake. You can either use a white pencil or use the lightest color in a makeup palette. It is also important to pair eyeshadow with red lips. It is good to go for dramatic red lips and cover unsightly blue lines on the lids with a concealer or shadow primer. Then keep the eyeshadow light. Whatever you do go for mineral makeup.

Let us take a look at mascara. The good thing about mascara is it does not clump, there is no need to use a lash comb for separation, it lengthens lashes, and it does not come off with water. Unfortunately, it has a tendency to flake and it goes on wet so it has the ability to come off initially on the lids. Overall, it goes on light and it separates lashes.

Let us talk about foundations and tinted moisturizers. If you want to cover up rosacea you need a yellow-tinted sheer tinted moisturizer. Don't use anything thicker because it will give you a masklike appearance. The yellow color will offset the red color. Don't use blush instead use a bronzer. The brown color in the bronzer offsets any redness in the cheeks. If you really want to have gorgeous skin, keep your skin healthy by cleansing, exfoliating, and hydrating the skin. Over time you won't need much concealer and you would probably use little foundation. It is also a good idea to slather on primer or a moisturizer before foundation. Applying concealer before foundation, avoiding full foundation coverage, blending the foundation the right way, picking the proper color and formula for the skin, using a brush, sponge, or fingers, never throw out wrong-tone foundations and concealers, concealing dark under-eye circles, having great highlighters, using bronzers, avoid "cake faces", using makeup with primers, using natural oils, using Evian spray, getting rid of a "ashen" look, toning down ruddy skin, creating nice cheeckbones, wear blush, and darken any ultra-white skin should all help make your skin look gorgeous.

Knowing how to apply blush can also enhance your beauty. Choosing a blush formulation is important. Blush comes in powder, gel, and cream forms. Creams work well on dry skin since it is blendable. General kind of powder is good to use on oily skin. Keep in mind Talc clogs the pores. You could use liquid and gel blushes for oily skin but they don't blend as well. Some of the women out there likes to combine both cream and powder together. This helps the blush stay on longer. First apply the cream and then the powder over it. Stains and gels should be put on to well-moisturized skin. They dry fast and they do a good job blending well and fast.

Choosing the color that is right for you is important. Use nature as a guide. Start looking for a shade that matches your cheek color when it is flushed from exercise or blushed from cold. Women with pink skin look best in pink shades. Women with olive or yellow skin tones look nice in peaches. Dark skin tones look great in apricot, red colors, or even dark pinks. It is good to match the lip color. It is good to try the product to see if it works before buying anything in a compact package.

When applying blush, start light and then build up. Apply a bit after foundation. Some people apply blush before foundation for a better natural look. Whenever applying blush, it is important to consider the shape of your face. Women who have long faces benefit applying blush to the apples of the cheeks. They then blend towards the hairline. Using C-shape shading can be used to apply blush to round or square shaped faces. Apply blush in a c-shape pattern from the temples to the cheekbones. It goes from the center of the brow bone to the center of the cheek. If you like to have a sun-kissed sheen, dab bronzer on the forehead, chin, and nose before applying blush. But be sure to use a large brush and a light hand. If you want to look sexy, dab a tiny bit of shimmery blush on your highest point of the cheekbone near the eye. Those who use cream or gel, use the middle finger to apply and then blend with the ring and middle finger. A clean finger can pick up any excess blush. Put a dot on the apple of the cheek and then put two smaller dots towards up the cheekbone. Then blend the dots all together all the way up to the hairline. Avoid using barbie-size makeup brushes. Use an actual blush brush. Brushes with real hair are good to use. It is also important to clean the brushes with baby wipes and then wash them with dish soap at least once a month. Dirty brushes accumulate bacteria and can be transferred to the skin. It is also important to apply blush the correct way. Place blush on the brush and then tap off excess or put a small dab of gel on the fingers. If you smile in front of a mirror, then this will help you figure out where the apple of the cheek is located. Put blush to the apples of the cheeks. If you use powder blush, sweep in only one direction. Do not go over and over or around and around because this causes streaks. It can also damage your brush. If for some reason you have gone over a bit heavy on the powder blush, use a bit of translucent powder to calm it down. If you are using a cream blush, choose to blot the color off with a tissue. The gel and liquid blush ends up staining the cheeks. If you want to lighten them, then wash your face. Moisturize and put the makeup again on. But do it sparingly. Finish with a look of your desire with a sweep of translucent powder.

Using eyeshadow primers such works well for eyeshadows. Use a good primer before putting on mascara. Some women put on moistrurizers before putting on makeup. Primers are better than moisturizers though. They help the makeup stay on longer and evens out skin tone. Foundation primers allow foundation to stay on during hot weather. It also helps the skin from absorbing talc and pigment from the foundation. It also prevents talc from drawing oil from the skin. Foundation primers also have botanicals such as aloe extracts, kiwi, geranium, grape, rose, jasmine, orange, and lavender. There are even nail and lip primers. They keep the lipstick and nail polish on longer and hopefully dry faster.

Picking the right shade of concealors is also important. Concealors do a good job transforming the skin tone. Concealors have the ability to cover up under-eye circles and blue veins under the eyes when the eyes are tired. When choosing a shade, go for a shade or 2 lighter than the skin. The foundation needs to match the skin tone. The only exception is when you are covering up pimples. Use a concealer that matches the skin exactly when you are covering up pimples. Apply the concealer after the foundation so you don't want the spot to stand out. Most women use a yellow-base concealer. It does a better job flattering the skin. Dark or black skin look better when using orange-based concealers. Under-eye concealers camouflages the shadowy circles under the eyes. Correctors cover up dark undereye circles. Yellow-toned concealers matches the skin tone exactly. Body concealers covers up veins on the legs. Heavy duty concealers cover up scars or other markings. When applying concealers, apply lots of dots of concealer under the eyes that is closest to the lashes. Even put a dot to the inside corners of the eyes. Using a concealer brush works better. But if you do not have it, you can use your finger. Use the pad of the brush and tap the concealer and blend it well. Apply the concealer on other spots that are uneven on the face. You may need to apply another layer for more coverage. Finally, dust fine and loose powder over the face to set the concealer.

Picking the perfect powder requires the work of trying out a few powders but do seek help from an associate. Mineral powders are better since they are natural products. If you choose the right powder it should disappear on the skin. Do not choose one that is lighter or darker than the skin. It is also a good idea to step outside or near a window to test the color itself. Never trust fluorescent lighting when putting on makeup. Keep in mind the quality of the brands are different between drugstores and department stores. Put a bit of powder under the eyes before applying eyeshadow. After applying the shadow, sweep away the powder itself using a tissue. Apply it with a fluffy makeup brush instead of a cushion-y pad. Again apply the powder after putting on other beauty products such as the concealer and foundation. Dip the brush inside the powder. Don't put powder all over the entire face. Use the brush and press it into the skin under the eyes. Then use it in a line from your forehead and then down the bridge of the nose to the chin.

Giving yourself a manicure can save both time and money. Some women feel the best nail shape is one that is not quite square and not quite oval. File nails into the shape that mirrors the curve of the nail base. If you want to make sure the nails are of the same length, line each of the nails with the counterparts. Do not shake the nail polish bottle. It is better to roll it between the palms. You can mix the polish better so that there are no air bubbles. Right before polishing clean nails, get a cotton ball, soak it in nail polish remover and swipe it across the nails. This removes excess oils or soap that causes peeling when the polish is applied. A good way to put nail polish is to hold the brush between the thumb and middle finger. At the same time rest the forefinger right on top of the cap.

If you want to get the best results, then apply it in thin layers. Start with a thin layer using a basecoat. Then apply a thin layer of polish down the middle and then one on the left and then one on the right. Let the first coat dry for a couple of minutes. Repeat it and then follow it with a thin layer of topcoat. Once the manicure is finished, use an orangewood stick that is dipped in nail polish remover along either side of the nails to fix mistakes. You can also speed up the drying process by using the blow-dryer at the toes. But make sure you set it at cool for about a minute. The dry should be about 12 inches from the feet. You can also apply cuticle oil over the nail polish. This keeps anything from sticking to the polish. Be sure you also remove stained nails. You can even use a damp towel from the microwave, put your feet in moisturizer and then wrap them in a warm towel.

Now the question we ask is how can we protect your manicure. Use a swipe of topcoat every other day on the manicure and about once a week on the pedicure. This will keep the polish from chipping. Using a nail buffer to help with chipped polish. You can repair a chip by smoothing any ragged edges with a buffer. It is then time to fill in the chip with polish. Wait until it is dry and then apply a coat over the entire nail. It is also not a good idea to file nails after a shower since they are very soft. It is better to file in one direction so that there won't be any tears.

If you are carrying out a pedicure, it is better to use a pedicure nail clipper for clipping toenails. Use a straight-edge since they won't allow the nails to be curved. Curved nails lead to painful ingrown nails. Slightly round the edges using a file. If you have a stubborn polish that ends up staining, put a cotton ball on the nail for many seconds before wiping it off. Putting more nail remover on the cotton makes the polish easier to remove. You can also protect your manicure by wearing gloves when carrying out indoor and outdoor tasks. If you are worried about dry cuticles, then use cuticle oil since it has more of an effect than creams.

So now you did your manicure. Let us take a look at pedicures. Exfoliate in the shower with a pumice stone in order to get rid of dead skin. Use a thick lotion or a cream to the feet. Once you are finished, wear socks when going to bed. If you really want extra soft feet, use a thick coat of diaper rash cream and put it on the feet. Then put the feet in a thin plastic bag and then put socks over it. Just make sure you don't make a mess while going to sleep by tossing and turning. If successful, then when you wake up in the morning you will have very soft feet. When growing nails, it is best not to grow out nails over an eighth to a quarter inch past the tips of the fingers. Have fun using neutral colors on the fingernails and a wide variety of colors on the feet.

Let us now take a look at fixing cracked cuticles. Winter season is a time when women get cracked cuticles. There seems to be a lack of moisture. You can also get cracked cuticles due to very dry skin or from washing hands too much. You can use a Vitamin E oil or shea butter in the cuticles so they can be soft. Another option is to use a super-strength cream on the hands and sleep in gloves during bedtime for a few days. You can also keep cuticle oil or cream nearby if you need it. Ingredients such as jojoba, sweet almond oils, and Vitamin E do a good job moisturizing the nail bed. Argan oil is probably the best cuticle oil out there. Use 100% on your cuticles at night or after washing your hands. It also works really well on dry heels and elbows as well.

French manicures are widely popular today. The first thing to do is to wash your hands and remove old nail polish. Use an acetone-free polish remover if the nails have a light shade. An acetone remover can be used for darker shades. Use an orangewood stick that has a covered end covered in cotton and dip it into the nail polish remover for the edges if this is needed. The next step is to clip the nails. Make a "squoval" shape which means the shape should not be a square or an oval. Clip the nails straight across. Get a file and file it in one direction. The corners should be slightly rounded. The next step is to prepare the nails. Take time to apply cuticle remover to cuticles. Place a few drops of jojoba or almond oil in a bowl that has a warm water. Soak the hands for a few minutes in the warm water and then pat the hands dry. Twist a portion of a water-moistened cotton on one end of an orangewood stick. Use the stick to push back the cuticles. Make sure you do not cut the cuticles. You risk the chance to nick the skin. Exfoliate the hands with a body scrub. Take time to rinse your hands and put hand cream. Then soak a cotton ball in a nail polish remover and swipe it across the nails. This removes the hand cream and extra oils or soap that could cause peeling when the polish is applied on the nails. Other nail shapes are also common.

UV penetration into the layers of the skin

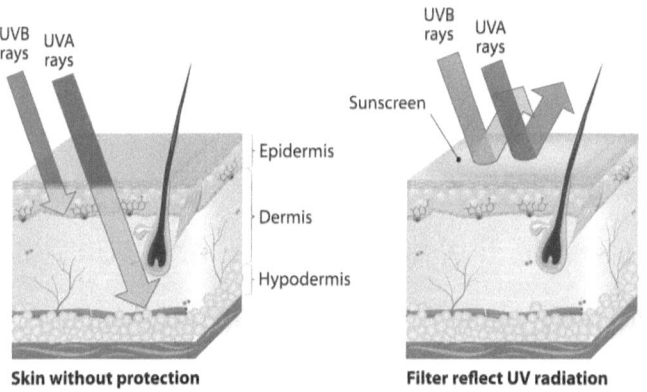

Skin without protection

Filter reflect UV radiation

The next step is to paint the nails. You need two shades of color. One of the colors is for the nail, and the other one is for the tip. You can choose neutral shades or shades with bright colors. Again remember that thin layers work the best. Make sure you do not shake the nail polish bottle. Roll the bottle between the palms. Mix the polish without causing air bubbles to form. Hold the brush between the thumb and middle finger. At the same time, rest your forefinger on the top of the cap. To begin with, start with a thin layer of basecoat to the pinky finger and then to the rest of the fingers. Put a thin layer of main polish down the middle, then a layer to the left, and then a layer to the right. Let the first coat dry and then repeat the procedure. Next comes painting the tip of the nail. Your nails can appear longer if you let the polish curve with the natural nail. Brush the polish over the edge and then wrap the polish under the nail. This prevents nails from chipping. Use an orange stick wrapped in cotton and moistened with polish remover to clean up any mess. Finish the French Manicure by applying a thin layer of a topcoat.

Let us now take a look at getting some of the best pedicures out there. The first step is to remove all nail polish. Use a lint-free cotton pad, saturate it, and rub it off the old polish. Nail polish remover that has alcohol-free and acetone-free removers work better on lighter nail polish shades. Then cut and file the nails. If you want to avoid ingrown nails, cut the nails straight across above the skin. Just make sure the nail does not extend over the tip of the toe. If you want to get a soft square shape, file the nails in one direction. They have to be slightly rounded at the corners and they have to be even. Metal files will only rip the nails. Using the Mehaz ingrown toenail file allows to life nail corners for better shaping. It is also not a good idea to clip the sides of the nails that causes ingrowns. Fine-grade surface is good for smoothing nail edges. The coarser surface is good for shortening and shaping nails. Then go ahead and soak your feet. Get a large bowl and fill it with warm water. Put bath salts and an aromatherapy oil and soak the feet for at least ten minutes. If you have more cracked and calloused feet, the longer they need to be stayed inside the warm water. If you add a quarter of milk to the bowl bath that helps even more. The lactic acid in milk loosens any dead skin present. The next step is to take care of the cuticles. Put cuticle remover towards the base of each nail and then rub it in. Leave the cuticle remover on for at least a minute. Use an orangestick to push using a circular motion where the skin meets the nails. Be cautious to remove the skin only on top of the nail. Make sure you do not touch the toe flesh. Be very careful you do not cut yourself if you use cuticle nippers to trim loose skin. Next scrub your feet. Use an exfoliating body or foot scrub to a wet pumice stone to remove dead skin on the balls and heels of the feet. Scrub the balls, bottom, and sides of the heels around the toes. Make sure you don't scrub too hard otherwise the skin can turn red. Next go ahead and moisturize your feet. Take the time to dry the feet thoroughly which includes between the toes and rub a thick moisturizer or perhaps a foot cream. Massage using the moisturizer into the feet and the calves. You can even rehydrate cuticles by rubbing a dab of cuticle oil. Then polish your toenails. You can use acetone remover to get rid of extra oils on the nails. Put a thin base coat using three strokes. Start with one down the middle and then one on each side. Make sure you don't paint the cuticle. Wait for at least a minute. Then add two coats of polish. Finish it off with a thin top coat. You probably have to clean up error using an orangestick that is wrapped in cotton and dipped in nail polish remover. Make sure you let your toenails dry for at least 45 minutes. A good technique when painting toenails is to paint remaining polish on the brush towards the front nail edge. This should prevent chipping. Once your nails are dried, then apply moisturizing oil all over your feet.

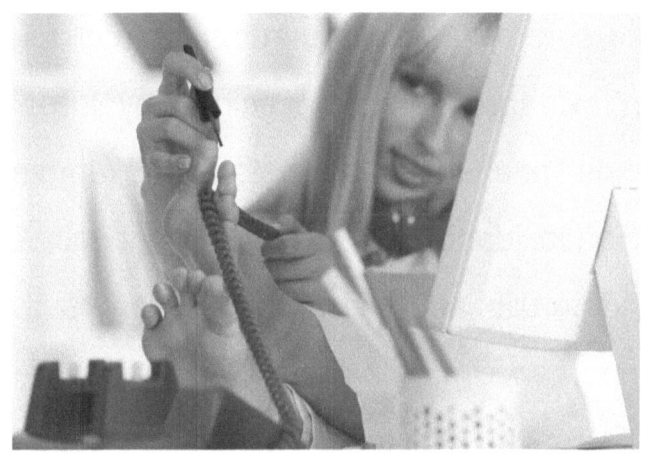

After having discussed both manicures and pedicures, let us take a look at some of the hottest nail trends. Some of the hottest nail trends are The Moon Manicure, Nail Tattoos, The Newsprint Manicure, Shatter Nail Polish, Shellac Polish, Gradual Ombre, Magnetic Nail Polish, Sports Nails, Rhinstones, Lace Nails, and Pointy Nails.

Let us talk about some of the best sunscreens out there in the market. It is good to have a sunscreen, retinol cream, and a skin serum. Good skin serums add moisture, antioxidants, glycolic acids, hyaluronic acids, and anti-inflammatories. Examples of antioxidants are Vitamin E, Vitamin C, and ferulic acid. They help improve the appearance of sun that damaged the skin and uneven skin tone. Vitamin C is good to use when used under sunscreen. Glycolic acid is used as a mild exfoliant. It breaks down dead skin cells and helps create new cells. The skin should be smoother. Hyaluronic acid is good for dry and aging skin. It boosts the skin's ability to retain moisture. Plants and nut-base oils adds moisture to the skin.

Some people ask if hair removal actually works. Let us take a look at some facts to see if laser hair removal is really for you. Both lasers and pulsed light ends up working best for people that have dark hair and light skin. But you need to be careful. Lasers can cause discoloration for those people with dark or tanned skin. Lasers are still under development as technology changes. You would need to ask if the salon's lasers will work for you or not. Lasers are powerful. They use pulse light to target and then break down melanin in hair. It works on dark hair. But they also target melanin in dark skin that can cause discoloration. Hair is known to grow in three phases. These phases include growing, resting, and shedding. Hair has a tendency to fall out in about 10-14 days. You can use a mild sugar scrub inside the shower on the tenth day. This can help exfoliate the skin and then remove the hair.

Laser and other forms of pulsed lights have the ability to target several follicles. This has the ability to treat large areas of the skin. Lasers can remove hair in under two hours. They are great for treating the back, shoulders, arms, and chests. When it comes to the upper lip and chin, lasers ends up working best on dark hair. Electrolysis works betters on blonde hairs. Keep in mind the treatments take long. It can take about 4-6 laser hair removal session that is spaced about 4 weeks apart if you want to see the majority of the hair to be reduced.

Keep in mind that laser hair removal does not work on all people. Hair does grow back for some people. Make sure you prepare for laser hair removal. Shave the day before the treatment or about three days before. When going through laser hair removal, you may find some areas may hurt and some areas may not hurt depending on the person. Some health professionals recommend to numb the skin about 20 minutes before the laser hair removal session with a spray or cream that has about 4% lidocaine. If you are going to get your hair removed, then find a qualified dermatologist or a licensed technician.

Let us take a look at shaving. The skin should soften before shaving. Do not shave dry skin. If you want to avoid nicks and cuts, then wet the skin and let it soften from both heat and moisture. Shaving can be thought of as a natural exfoliator. If you dry shave, you may end up clogging the razor with dead skin and you may end up getting nicks and razor burns. It seems to me the shaving creams for women work just as good for the shaving creams for men. It is good to apply baby oil before using the shaving cream. If you want to avoid burn in the shower, then put on baby oil in the tub to make sure you soften the skin. Then put on the shaving cream. Oil and water do not mix. The oil will stay on throughout the time you are in the shower. You might be able to avoid both nick- and razor-burn free with soft legs. If you don't have anymore shaving cream, then you can use olive oil to shave the legs. Hair conditioner works for shaving since it is moisturizing. Shampoo tends to dry. When using a razor get the one with lubricated strips, pivoting heads, and spring-mounted multiple blades. Never use a dull razor and never share a razor with someone else. You could catch a disease. Make sure you exfoliate before shaving. You want to get rid of the dead skin cells so the razor does not get clogged. Use exfoliating gloves or maybe a cloth inside the shower or a dry brush before you take a shower.

Shaving the proper way is important. Leg hairs grow down. Start at the ankles and then shave up. If you shave the underarms, then you will need to shave in all directions. Hair grows in several different angles. When you are shaving your legs, use the razor on each spot twice. First shave against hair growth and then shave in the direction the hair is growing. This gives the hair a pointed tip to make it grow out in a nice fashion. After you are done shaving, put oil or a moisturizer. The skin only has a few glands and can dry. You can also avoid ingrown hairs by exfoliating on a daily basis. Use a glycolic acid cleanser on the affected areas.

It may also be better to wax on the bikini line and lower legs. Use the razor for the underarms and upper legs.

Waxing or sugaring gets rid of bikini hair. Both of them work better to get rid of bikini hair. Waxing involves putting it on the skin. The resin binds to the hair to a strip of cloth. The cloth is then removed in the opposite direction where the hair is growing. The hair is removed from the roots but in time they grow back. Sugaring is an alternative form to wax. It is made of a mixture of lemon juice, sugar, and water. The hair needs to be long for the waxing to take place. The wax needs to bind to the hair in order to be pulled out. You can also use a paste and apply it with the hands instead of using a stick. Another sugaring method is to use a gel and apply it the same way as a wax.

The legs and bikini are good spots for both waxing and sugaring. The upper lips and brows are also good spots. Even some people get their arms waxed or sugared. Back waxings on males have also become common. Keep in mind these processes are painful but in time you might get used to it. Waxing and sugaring can last up to two to six weeks.

It is also important to use moisturizers to avoid dry skin during the winter. Low temperatures and low humidity along with strong winds reduces the skin's natural lipid layer. It keeps the skin from drying. Dry hair from heating sources also take moisture out of the skin. You want to keep the skin soft by keeping moisture in it. You want to keep the water lukewarm. Do not use hot water since it removes moisture from the skin and causes it to dry. Take a shower in lukewarm water. Wash hands also in lukewarm water. Use moisturizers after taking a shower or washing the hands. Oils adds moisture to the skin and when that is soaked in, apply a layer of cream. When you are cleaning the face, use an oil cleanser.

It is also a good idea to exfoliate either on a weekly or semi-weekly basis. Exfoliation involves the removal of old dead skin cells on the skin's outermost surface. It is involved when facials are carried out such as microdermabrasion or chemical peels. Chemical exfoliants include specific scrubs that contain salicylic acid, glycolic acid, fruit enzymes, malic acid, or even citric acid. These chemicals can be applied in high concentrations by medical professionals or in lower concentrations from over-the-counter products. Chemical exfoliation can also include products containing alpha hydroxy acids or AHAs, beta hydroxyacids or BHAs or enzymes that loosen cells together. This type of exfoliation is useful for people treating acne. Even AHAs are known to reduce wrinkles and signs of aging.

But when it comes to moisturizers, they are better on exfoliated skin. You may want to use a salt ot sugar scrub while in the shower and then exfoliate the face with a mild scrub that is made with the face at least one time per week. You could apply coconut oil on the cleansed face, and then use a warm and wet washcloth to massage the oil inside the skin. This tends to exfoliate and moisturize. Apply it on the body and then add sugar or salt to the oil to make your scrub. You can also dry brush the skin before you take a shower. This helps relieve dry skin. Humidifiers can be good to use if you live in a low-humidity climate or if you are around furnaces during the winter. The skin needs to be more than 30% humidity in order to stay moisturized. During the winder, sleep with a humidifier in your own bedroom and make sure the doors are closed so air does not escape.

Taking care of the face is also important. Use special cleansers and masks that is formulated for the face. It is not a good idea to cleanse the face using a body soap. Soaps have the ability to dry. You may want to use a creamy moisturizer cleanser that has glycerin or petrolatum. For the hands put moisturizer and gloves on before going outdoors in the winter. Put moisture on the feet and sleep in cotton socks at night time. It is also a good idea keep the feet soft. Cover the feet with a thick moisturizer and then wrap the feet in Saran Wrap. Then put on a pair of socks for a couple of hours. Take time to lie down while the moisturizer soaks in. When it comes to moisturizing your lips, do not lick them. They will eventually dry out. Lips have less moisture than other parts on our bodies. Using lip balm helps the lips to be moisturized. When it comes to the face, avoid using tap water. Tap water has harsh minerals that dry the skin. It might be better to use cold cream to clean the face or use spring water. Omega-3 fish oil pills can soothe dry skin. Omega-6 fatty acids are found in grains, oils from plants, and eggs. Omega-3 fatty acids are found in cold-water fish such as salmon and tuna.

Removing makeup requires proper steps. You need a cleanser for the face and a eye makeup remover. Soak soft cotton pads or balls in a eye makeup remover. Let them sit atop of the eyes for a few seconds. This should be able to loosen the makeup without even scrubbing. Always pat and never rub when it comes to the eyes. Fine lines will develop anyway. Eye makeup removers are better when removing makeup. As for the lips, remove any lip color before cleansing the face. You don't want to smear lipstick over the cleansed face. If you want to remove makeup on the face, use a cream or oil cleansers. If you have oily or a combination skin, use a cleanser that is formulated for your own skin type. You should also wash the face before going to bed if you have makeup and sunscreen on the face. In the morning, put a bit of warm water on the face so the oils can dissolve. Put a warm washcloth on the face. Using toner to remove makeup ends up stripping the skin and removes natural oils which leads to drying. Baby wipes should not be used to remove makeup. You want to remove makeup without drying it out even more. Again choose a cleanser based on what kind of skin you have. A cleansing oil can be used if you have super dry skin. Put oil on a cotton pad and swipe the oil across the lids, lips, face, and brows. Massaging the oil ends up loosening dirt and makeup. Wash the skin with a foam cleanser, and then wash off the cleanser with a warm washcloth. This ends up exfoliating the skin. Apply the moisturizer to dampen the skin. If you have acne, wash the face with salicylic cleanser. If your skin is oily, use a foaming cleanser.

"Cleansing your face is the most important part of your home care skin regime. You will need to use a cleanser that is formulated for the skin type (oily, dry, combination, normal) "and condition" i.e. acni, dry, dehydrated, sensitized, roacea, etc.." (from Christal Petrak)

Rinse the face and neck with lukewarm water. Put the cleanser on the forehead, chin, cheeks, and neck. Massage the cleanser on the face and neck in a circular motion for about a minute. Make sure you don't forget the nose and chin. Rinse the face and neck with a warm washcloth. Make sure you remove eye makeup with a makeup remover. The second step is to exfoliate. Use a facial scrub and exfoliate in a circular motion on the face. Use your fingers and work on the area around the nose and forehead. You may need to work harder on areas that tend to be greasy. Then use a soft washcloth that is soaked in warm water in order to rinse the face. The washcloth is used as a natural exfoliant. The third step is to use steam. Fill the sink with warm water, then dip a washcloth inside, and then press it to the face and then repeat it two times. The fourth step is to put a mask. If you have oil skin, use a clay-based face mask. If you have dry skin, use a hydrating gel or cream mask. Put the mask on and avoid the areas surrounding the eyes. Keep the mask on for about 10-20 minutes. The last step is to use a moisturizer. Put a moisturizer on the face and neck.

Using the right scrub is important. Sugar scrubs to drying salt scrubs work good.

Cheap scrubs have granules that micro-tear the skin. Other scrubs have microbeads that are not good for the environment because they are too small to be filtered out of water treatment plants after being washed down sinks. The beads go to the oceans and lakes and they are not biodegradable.

Use either a bath mit or bath gloves when using a scrub. You can even put them in the washing machine and let them air dry. Dry brushing exfoliates the skin and lets the lymphatic system drain waste. When you use a dry brush that means you do not use water. It is also not a good idea to keep the wooden brush in the hot bathroom. It can become a mold collector. You have to remain naked and get into the shower. Start at your feet and brush the skin from the toes to the top of the thighs. Use short and swift brush strokes. Move towards the heart. Go over the same places but do it in slow circular motions. Brush from the stomach to the chest. Move to the arms by going from the fingertips to the shoulders. Brush the skin on the buttocks from the bottom to the top. Brush the lower back towards the shoulders. Then take a shower and apply moisturizer. Give it about a month and you should be able to see a difference. The skin should be softer.

When you are scrubbing start at the feet and massage the scrub in circular motions to the legs and torso. Continue to the fingertips and massage up to the arm. Do not over exfoliate and just scrub a couple times a week. Use a lighter touch if you have sensitive skin. Do not scrub after shaving. You can sting the skin. Use a good scrub before shaving which removes dead skin cells. This will help prevent clogging the razor. Put on oil after taking a bath. A thick moisturizer or oil should work. Do apply moisturizer after scrubbing.

Taking care of the feet is just as important as any other part of the body. Soak the feet for at least 15 minutes inside a warm foot bath. The foot bath should consist of a cup of milk and a decent size volume of warm water. The longer you spend time soaking in the warm water bath, the skin has more time to soften. You will then be able to scrub away the dead bits. Use a foot scrub and massage it in a circular motion into the bottoms of the feet. Then use a pumice stone or a lava stone to scrub the feet. Take time to rinse and dry the feet. Use a Stridex pad, which contains 2% salicylic acid, to rub over dry areas of the feet. This pad has the ability to exfoliate dead skin, and it works nicely on the feet. Let the Stridex dry and do not wash it off. Put a super-rich foot cream on the feet and go to sleep wearing socks. The next night put a thin layer of salicylic acid cream on the feet and a dollop of Vaseline. Again sleep with the socks on. Hopefully, this procedure should give you excellent results.

Washclothes are good for exfoliating the face. Put cleanser on the face. Take a wash cloth and wet it. Massage the cleanser into the skin in circular motions. Rinse the face. If you want some extra exfoliating benefits, then sprinkle some sugar into the cleanser before massaging it on the skin. Then use a warm and damp washcloth to remove the cleanser. You can also reduce puffiness using a washcloth that is soaked in ice water. Put the cold washcloth on the face and then hold it for a few seconds. Women who are over 35 years old have oily skin underneath and dry skin on the surface. You will need to examine the skin before putting makeup on if you are concerned about flakiness. If there are flakes, put a dry washcloth over the face. It should erase the flakes. Then put moisturizer before putting on foundation or some tinted moisturizer. You can even shave the legs using a washcloth. Wet your hands and put either soap or shaving cream. Then go ahead and shave the legs. Then use a warm wet washcloth over the legs and rinse off the cream. Take time to rinse and repeat the process as many times as needed.

If you want to exfoliate flaky lips, then use a damp washcloth. Rub the lips in a circular motion using a damp washcloth before putting on gloss or a lip balm. Put a warm washcloth into sugar if you need extra exfoliating. It is also better to use washcloths in the shower than shower poufs since they have less bacteria. Take time to change yours everyday. At night time, wet a washcloth in hot water and wring it out. Put it on the face until the washcloth cools down. Then put moisturizer on. Use a quick exfoliant before putting tanner on the legs. Use a leg shimmer and rub the legs with a dry washcloth. Then put the self-tanner on the skin. Do a quick wash of there is no time for a shower. You can use a washcloth to wash spots that normally needs to be clean. Anti-aging and age-management is important to a lot of people especially women. Instringic, extringic, prevention, spf protection, antioxidants, and hydration are all factors that should be considered.

Some people feel Retin-A (tretinoin) is a prescrition drug that works for anti-aging. It is not a cosmetic. Tretinoin reduces fine lines and wrinkles. It is a derivative of Vitamin A. Taking care of the collagen is the secret to a healthy skin. It tends to age well. A change in the pH level of the skin by using a Vitamin A product like Retin-A helps generate collagen. If you want to avoid keeping collagen from breaking down, then avoid the sun. Most wrinkles, dark spots, and sun damage have to do with too much sun exposure. This is why it is best to use sunscreen. It is not a good idea to expose the skin to the sun whenever you use retinols. It is better to cover up with sunscreen and wear a hat. Vitamin A has the ability to make the skin susceptible to skin damage. It is also not a good idea to use tretinoin products if you are currently pregnant. If you decide to use this product, be very careful. It can cause redness, peeling, and flaking. Some women use it twice a week and then slowly move to every other day. This gives time for the skin to adjust. As mentioned, the skin can become irritated using Retin-A. If the skin becomes dry and reddened, then stop using the skincare and apply extra virgin oil during nightime before going to bed. Olive oil has fatty acids and is therefore a good moisturizer.

Alpha hydroxy acids are derived from natural products such as sugar, cane, tomatoes, and milk. They are used as mild exfoliants. They break down dead skin cells and create new cells. Alpha hydroxy acids are made from food products which include glycolic acid (sugar cane), lactic acid (sour milk), malic acid (apples), citric acid (citrus fruits), and tartaric acid (grape wine). Milder creams should be used every day. The skin complexion improves, gets smoother, and has fewer blackheads. Alpha hydroxy acids are found in topical creams, scrubs, and moisturizers. It is best to avoid alpha hydroxy acids if your skin is sensitive or if you have to spend a lot of time in the sun. You become susceptible to sunburn whenever you use alpha hydroxy acids. ALWAYS use a high SPF sunscreen on the face and wear a hat when you are in the sun when using AHA's. Antioxidant serums work just like vitamins and can be used on the skin. Free radicals which are unstable oxygen molecules cause skin problems. These radicals attack healthy skin cells. They even cause collagen to breakdown which then leads to wrinkles. You can protect yourself from free radicals by using an antioxidant cream preferrably to use in the morning. Make sure it has the ingredients green tea, Vitamins C and E, and Coenzyme Q10. The molecules work together to neutralize free radicals. Be careful choosing products that promise too much because most of the time the product does not necessarily give the best results. Products based on scientific results are more promising and are normally considered to be professional products. Over the counter products are usually not scientific tested and the consumer assumes a greater risk of adverse side effects.

Combating Wrinkles as women get older is common. Dry skin, UV exposure, oxidated stress ends up leading to wrinkles. It is best to use a moisturizer. As mentioned, retinoids and retinol might work but caution should be used. Alpha hydroxy acids also work as well. But I have not had a chance to talk more about antioxidants. They also help with UV protection. As mentioned before, sun damage causes wrinkles. Lighter skin are more susceptible wrinkles when exposed to the sun. Wear at least an SPF 30 sunscreen to prevent the skin from being damaged. It is best to look for sunscreen that has both UVA and UVB protection. Let us take a look at hydroquinone. It is an aromatic compound with two hydroxyl groups oriented in the para position. It is known to be a human respiratory toxicant and a allergen. Dark spots found on the skin may be caused by sun damage, hormones, environmental stress, acne, etc. They make the skin appear older than it really is. A hydroquinone cream could also be used. Apply it to dark spot at nighttime. It could take a few weeks for their to be positive results. There are other basic ways to keep your skin in good shape. We should all get plenty of rest. Some women like to wear sunglasses, hat, and long sleeves when it is sunny outside. Stress can also leads to wrinkles. Some women like to do meditation or yoga to relieve stress such as soaking with Epsom and Dead Sea Salts.

Maybe you might want to put a UVA/UVB protector screen on your driver's side of the car window if you drive a lot. Lines form more on the left face for those who drive a lot. A high-quality cleanser should rinse off easily with water. Even the toners make pores look smaller by swelling the tissue around the pore, a moisturizer can have the same effect and do more.

Wrinkles can be reduced with a chocolate waste product. There are antioxidants benefits of cocoa pods in a anti-wrinkle gel. These pods contain antioxidant compounds such as malic acid, procandidin B1, rosmarinic acid, procyanidin C1, ellagic acid, and apigenin. Skin wrinkles improved and skin hydration increased. Cocoa pod extract may very well be an ingredient for future cosmetic products.

Ubiquinone or coenzyme Q10 and idebenone are antioxidants that have been reported to be effective for the skin. The molecules protect our skin from oxidation caused by pollution and ultraviolet irradiation. This helps the skin from premature aging.

Curcumin combined with niacinamide has shown results against the appearance of wrinkles and fine lines.

Sesame oil referred to as the "the golden serum" has Vitamin E, palmitic acids, linoleic acids, and the antioxidant sesamol is a natural moisturizer and emollient. All of these antioxidants gives healing from the sun and damages from the wind. It slows the premature aging process. It does this by slowing cell growth and the process of replication. It also soothes and protects our skin. It is also used for irritation and dandruff. It protects us from the sun and chlorine. Sesame oil binds dirt, toxins, and oils. Quercetin is a bioflavinoid. It is a plant pigment that gives fruits, flowers, and vegetable their color. Flavinoids are antioxidants and get rid of free radicals which damages cell membranes. Quercetin protects the skin from UVA radiation.

Rutin is a plant bioflavinoid found in citrus fruits, vegetables, leaves, and grains. It has the ability to regenerate Vitmain C after neutralizing free radicals. This makes it an excellent antioxidant. Both rutin and quercetin inhibit collagen from breaking down. It is also antiinflammatory. The Mirabilis jalapa plant or the "Marvel of Peru" has shown potential to treat sensitive and reactive skin. This plant may have the ability to combat inflammation and problems such as rosacea and hypersensitive skin.

Let us talk about essential oil chemistry. Terpenes are hydrocarbons that discharge toxins from the kidneys and liver. They also inhibit the accumulation of toxins. Sesquiterpenes are known to be antiseptic and anti-inflammatory. They help cellular memory and they are found in essential oils. Easter are formed from reactions of an alcohol with an acid. They are found in a large number of oils. They are considered to be anti-fungal. They also have calming and relaxing effects. The functional group aldehydes are reactive and are anti-infectious. They have a sedative effect on the central nervous system. It is possible they can cause irritation or dermatitis. But when they are inhaled, they have a calming effect. Ketones give cellular regeneration which then promotes tissue formation and liquify mucous. They are found in oils for the upper respiratory system. Alcohols are known for the antiseptic and anti-viral activities. They have the ability to create uplifting quality. They are also nontoxic.

Phenols are antiseptic, antibacterial, and they can be stimulating. They could cause skin sensitivity if they are undiluted. But they do have antioxidant properties.

Let me conclude with some tips on healthy skin. If your skin is exposed to a lot of sun, smoke, and stress, then your skin can starting looking old.

Aged Skin Section

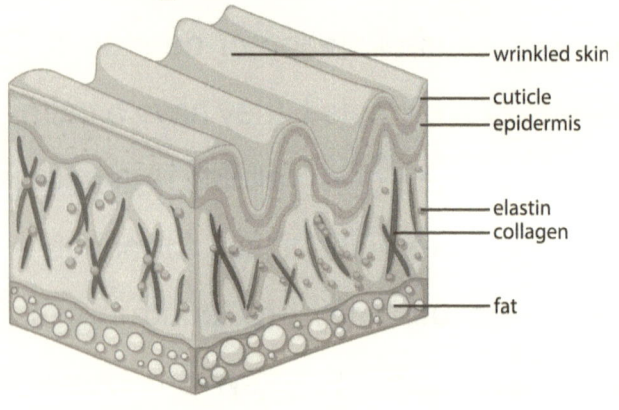

It does this because it loses its collagen, but keep in mind the process is still more complex. Both the glow and elasticity is gone. Lines could develop prematurely. The skin will also start looking dull. Make sure you don't smoke, if you want to keep that youthful glow in your skin.

"Smoking especially second hand smoke is the worst thing you can do for your skin, next to not cleansing off your makeup before bed", according to Christal Petrak.

Nicotine has the ability to constrict blood vessels and then decrease the flow of oxygen to the skin. Using a retinoid lotion is an anti-aging lotion that works, but it needs to be used with caution. Getting regular facials will also help. Wearing sunscreen will help too. Window shields for cars with SPF 285 has the ability to block UVA and

UVB rays. It is not a good idea to pull and rub the skin. UV rays, stress, and carbon monoxide attacks the aging skin. Never skip moisturizing the face. Wrinkles are formed by dry skin. Moisturizers improve any lines on the face. Do not forget to take care of the neck and chest. Both the neck and chest have fewer oil glands than other parts of the body. They show signs of aging. Unfortunately most people ignore them Choose moisturizers that have the ingredients Vitamin A, copper, kinetin, and Vitamin C. These ingredients fight against aging. If you want to appear younger, do not tan. Tanning will cause wrinkles. It can get very costly to take care of yourself when signs of aging appears. But if you do have sun damage to your skin, it can be reversed by photorejuvenation. Pulsed light treatments work but again they are expensive. Some women feel it is cheaper to use lemon juice diluted with water to treat brown spots. Using a Q-tip and dipping it in the mixture at least twice a day might make the sun spots fade. Finally, take care of the skin on a daily basis. Cleaning the face every night can help avoid clogged pores and wash away any dirt and pollution. Anti-aging products needs to be used cautiously. You may suffer redness and some peeling to begin with. However, this is normal. If you want to get the best effects of acid peels, alpha hydroxy acids, retinoids, and moisturizers you have to keep using it. Check with your skincare professional on the best facial treatments and skincare products to best suite your skin issues or specific needs.

Dead sea salts have benefits when taking care of the skin. The Dead Sea is dense, and it is known to be a body of water over 1,000 feet below sea level. It is one of the lowest places on earth. It is located in both Israel and Jordon. It is also more saltier than the rest of the ocean since both plants and animals don't live there. Dead sea salts contain of minerals that has benefits for the skin. Minerals such as magnesium, calcium, bromide, sulfur, potassium, sodium, and zinc are examples of Dead Sea salts. These salts help the skin hold onto water, and they also help the skin stay moisturized. Using the right kinds of salts actually hydrates the skin. Both water and salt including potassium regulates water content inside our cells. It delivers nutrients to cells, and it also helps remove toxins and metabolic wastes from cells. As water gets into cells, potassium is what keeps it there. We get potassium from fruits and vegetables. Salt's main role is to regulat water by keeping water outside the cells.

Both magnesium and calcium sometimes can make the skin's barrier stronger. There is more to it than that. Dead Sea salts give better circulation in the skin and speeds processes where old skin cells get replaced by new skin cells, improve skin roughness, and even reduce inflammation. They even can be anti-aging. You can relax your muscles and relieve stress by soaking in a bath full of Dead Sea salts. Some people soak in Dead Sea salts for at least 15-20 minutes and then apply a moisturizer. Furthermore, Dead Sea salts provide extra hydration. Thank you for taking the time to read "What You Need To Know About Complexion Perfecters" and I wish you the best in choosing the best cosmetic products that will continue to enhance your life and succeed.

Gold has recently been used in spa skin care for anti-aging and anti-inflammatory benefits. The microparticles have the ability to hydrate and firm the skin which in turn helps retain collagen. The particles get easily absorbed into the skin which then creates an instant glow. Moisture is also increased. Gold in treatment products increase skin cell metabolism and function. It reduces inflammation, breakouts and the skin becomes more firm and hydrated. Gold also reduces hyperpigmentation, used as an antibaterial agent, and antioxidizes the skin.

Micro silver has been used to reduce irritation and redness linked to rosacea and sensitive skin. It also helps with antimicrobial effects. The microscopic particle stick to the surface of the skin longer than silver powders. They rest in skin folds and release silver particles over time. Colloidal forms of silve can be used to soothe and heal the skin found in professional products containing silver. It can boost the skin's immune system and regenerate healthy skin. It has anti-inflammatory properties that soothes the skin.

Copper is a common ingredient used in professional skin care products. It is found in its peptide form for anti-aging effects. Copper has been used to reduce advanced glycation end-product formation as well as inflammation. They keep stem cells alive and enhance wound-healing and tissue regeneration. It can be combined with peptides to give renewal of the signs of aging. Copper peptides have also been used to improve the appearance of lash and brow hair. It provides protection against breakout and gives a youthful appearance of lashes and brows. Copper tripeptide-1 has also been used to increase collagen production for anti-aging. It has also been used to regulate sebum production in oily skin. Copper has been linked to protect against nature's stressors such as exhaust, smoke, ozone, and even free radicals that prematurely age, weaken, and ends up dehydrating and sensitizing the skin. Copper is definitely an important trace element that neutralizes the skin's ability to undergo oxidative stress. Research will continue to progress with new forms and formulations will still be carried out.

I like to conclude with the future of anti-wrinkle technology known as drone science. Drone science is known to target cells to fill wrinkles. They increase elastin synthesis. Encapsulated free peptides protect cells from dehydration. This technology has the power to reverse the suppression of HAS2 mRNA found in fibroblasts. It induces its expression to fill wrinkles which is one of the effective methods for treating the skin.

Remember there are six tips to stay young and reduce signs of aging. Don't eat too much, making love, keep learning a variety of things in life, reduce belly fat, eat more plant-rich foods, and drinking red wine as long as you are not allergic to plant-rich foods and red wine. Please do check with your doctor to see what would be best for you. I wish you the best to staying healthy, young, and living a great lifestyle knowing more about both cosmetics and chemistry.

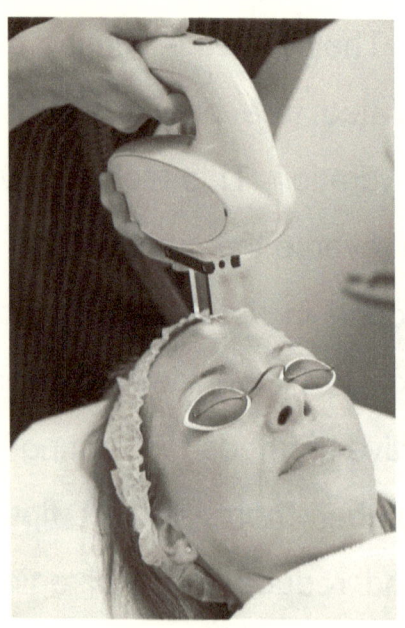

About the Author

Harminder Gill did his undergraduate studies at the University of California, Riverside, where he finished his bachelor of science degree in biological chemistry with an emphasis in chemistry. After completing his undergraduate studies, he attended graduate school at the University of California, Davis, where he finished his master's degree in organic chemistry. After doing several teaching assignments, he went into the teaching profession at community colleges. He was an adjunct professor at many community colleges in Southern California. He became a life member for both the alumni associations at

UCR and UCD. He has done homeschooling throughout communities, where he offers more than two hundred sections of academic subjects from humanities, social sciences, sciences, and test preparation. Plenty of his past students have done exceptionally well, including those who have achieved high scores on standardized tests, getting accepted into training academies, universities, and programs of their choice. He has served on board of directors, completed the distinguished toastmaster (DTM) in the Toastmasters Program for Public Speaking and Leadership, and he is currently a docent at museums and a science institute. He does his best to keep current in the math, sciences, and technology.

References

Voet, Donald and Voet, Judith G. Biochemistry Second Edition. John Wiley & Sons, Inc. 1995

Zumdahl, Steven S. and Zumdahl, Susan A. Chemistry Sixth Edition. Houghton Mifflon Company. 2003

Timberlake, Karen C. Ninth Edition. Benjamin Cummings. 2006.

http://www.skininc.com/treatments/

http://www.skininc.com/treatments/facial/

http://www.skininc.com/treatments/cosmetics/

http://www.skininc.com/skinscience/

http://www.skininc.com/skinscience/ingredients/

http://www.skininc.com/skinscience/physiology/

http://www.circadia.com

http://www.sterlingminerals.com/why-do-you-use-cosmetic-fillers-in-your-mineral-makeup/

https://www.organicconsumers.org/news/natural-consumer-products-found-contaminated-cancer-causing-14-dioxane-groundbreaking-analysis

http://guardianlv.com/2014/05/microbeads-in-face-wash-bad-for-the-environment/

http://www.ewg.org/skindeep/ingredient/703041/HYDROQUINONE/

http://www.waterbenefitshealth.com/water-and-salt.html

http://www.skininc.com/skinscience/ingredients/Precious-Metals-Skin-Loves-Gold-Silver-and-Copper-392775101.html

http://en.wikipedia.org/wiki/Cosmetics

http://en.wikipedia.org/wiki/Primer_(cosmetics)

http://en.wikipedia.org/wiki

Foundation_(cosmetics)

http://www.en.wikipedia.org/wiki/Facepowder

http://en.wikipedia.org/wiki/Rouge_(cosmetics)

http://www.wikihow.com/Apply-Bronzer

http://en.wikipedia.org/wiki/Mascara

http://naturalhealthtechniques.com/list-ofcosmetics.htm

http://www.chemistryexplained.com/CoDi/Cosmetic-
Chemistry.html#b

http://beauty.about.com/od/organic-skincare/ss/Organic-
Beauty-20-Things-You-Need-to-Know.htm,

http://beauty.about.com/od/bestcutsbyfaceshap1/ss/Are-
You-Round-Square-Long-Heart-Or-Oval.htm

http://beauty.about.com/od/bestcutsbyfaceshap1/ss/Are-
You-Round-Square-Long-Heart-Or-Oval.htm#step2

http://beauty.about.com/od/bestcutsbyfaceshap1/ss/Are-
You-Round-Square-Long-Heart-Or-Oval.htm#step3

http://beauty.about.com/od/bestcutsbyfaceshap1/ss/Are-
You-Round-Square-Long-Heart-Or-Oval.htm#step4

http://beauty.about.com/od/bestcutsbyfaceshap1/ss/Are-
You-Round-Square-Long-Heart-Or-Oval.htm#step5

http://beauty.about.com/od/bestcutsbyfaceshap1/ss/Are-
You-Round-Square-Long-Heart-Or-Oval.htm#step6

http://beauty.about.com/od/bestcutsbyfaceshap1/ss/Are-
You-Round-Square-Long-Heart-Or-Oval.htm#step7

http://beauty.about.com/od/eyeshadow/qt/eyeshad1.htm

http://beauty.about.com/od/mascara/gr/definicils.htm

http://beauty.about.com/od/eyeshadow/qt/eyeshad1.htm

http://beauty.about.com/od/allaboutyoureyes/a/
eyelinertips.htm

http://beauty.about.com/od/eyebrows/qt/sparsebrows.htm

http://beauty.about.com/od/makeuptrickstips/ht/
curllashes.htm

http://beauty.about.com/od/foundationsconcealers/f/
foundationhelp.htm

http://beauty.about.com/od/makeuptrickstips/ht/blush.htm

http://beauty.about.com/od/foundationsconcealers/f/
primer.htm

http://beauty.about.com/od/makeupbrushes/a/How-To-
Clean-Your-Makeup-Brushes.htm

http://beauty.about.com/od/makeuptrickstips/a/
beautrend.htm

http://beauty.about.com/od/concealers/qt/
concealershade.htm

http://beauty.about.com/od/powder/tp/Best-Pressed-And-
Loose-Powders.htm

http://beauty.about.com/od/eyeshadow/a/How-To-Fake-A-
Full-Night-Of-Sleep.htm

http://beauty.about.com/od/makeuptrickstips/a/shelflife.htm

http://beauty.about.com/od/lipbalm/fr/Review-Of-Burts-
Bees-Tinted-Lip-Balm.htm

http://beauty.about.com/od/lipstick/qt/fulllips.htm

http://beauty.about.com/od/lipstick/a/lipstick.htm

http://beauty.about.com/od/lipgloss/tp/
best_lip_glosses.htm

http://beauty.about.com/od/celebrityfragrances/

http://beauty.about.com/od/celebrityfragrances/tp/top-10-
celebrity-fragrances.htm

http://beauty.about.com/od/fragranc1/a/different-types-of-
perfume.htm

http://beauty.about.com/od/bestfragrancesbyseason/tp/
best-summer-perfumes-2011.htm

http://beauty.about.com/od/fragranc1/tp/best-winter-perfumes-and-fragrances-2010.htm

http://beauty.about.com/od/fragranc1/tp/top-10-perfumes-for-spring-2011.htm

http://beauty.about.com/od/eyeshadow/tp/Natural-Eye-Makeup.htm

http://beauty.about.com/od/mascara/ss/Mascara-The-13-Best-Mascaras-of-2015.htm

http://beauty.about.com/od/foundationsconcealers/a/foundtips.htm

http://beauty.about.com/od/concealers/qt/concealerapply.htm

http://beauty.about.com/od/powder/qt/How-To-Properly-Apply-Face-Powder.htm

http://beauty.about.com/od/celebrityfragrances/tp/top-10-celebrity-fragrances.htm

http://beauty.about.com/od/fragranc1/a/different-types-of-perfume.htm

http://beauty.about.com/od/fragranc1/a/review-of-joy-perfume.htm

http://beauty.about.com/od/bestfragrancesbyseason/tp/best-summer-perfumes-2011.htm

http://beauty.about.com/od/fragranc1/tp/top-10-perfumes-for-spring-2011.htm

http://beauty.about.com/od/fragranc1/a/popular-fragrance-terms.htm

http://beauty.about.com/od/faketanners/a/How-To-Tan-Your-Skin-Safely.htm

http://beauty.about.com/od/laserhairremoval/a/laserfacts.htm

http://beauty.about.com/od/hairremoval/a/shavetips.htm

http://beauty.about.com/od/hairremoval/f/waxingsugaring.htm

http://beauty.about.com/od/skinflaws/a/skinsavers.htm

http://beauty.about.com/od/makeuptrickstips/qt/removemakeup.htm

http://beauty.about.com/od/bathtime/qt/scrubs1.htm

http://beauty.about.com/od/dryskinfixes/ht/dry_cracked_heels.htm

http://beauty.about.com/od/plasticsurger1/a/5-Amazing-Uses-For-Botox.htm

http://beauty.about.com/od/beautybyageteensto50/g/peelswhat.htm

http://beauty.about.com/od/skinflaws/a/retinoids.htm

http://beauty.about.com/od/skinflaws/a/agingskin.htm

http://skincare.about.com/od/Skin-Care-Ingredients/fl/Dead-Sea-Salts-Can-Save-Your-Skin.htm?utm_campaign=stylensl&utm_medium=email&utm_source=cn_nl&utm_content=7781193&utm_term=bouncex11

http://www.skininc.com/treatments/cosmetics/19070719.html?utm_source=Most+Read&utm_medium=website&utm_campaign=Most+Read

http://www.skininc.com/skinscience/ingredients/Reduce-Wrinkles-With-a-Chocolate-Waste-Product-376557561.html

http://www.skininc.com/skinscience/ingredients/Ingredient-Insights-CoQ10-Idebenone-and-Curcumin-371414721.html

http://www.skininc.com/skinscience/ingredients/Liquid-Gold-The-Power-of-Plant-Oils-338843592.html

http://www.skininc.com/skinscience/ingredients/Natural-Anti-inflammatory-Ingredients-320276471.html

http://www.skininc.com/skinscience/ingredients/The-Science-of-Essential-Oils-303299761.html

http://www.health.com/health/gallery/0,,20356118,00.html#pour-yourself-some-merlot-0

www.ingramcontent.com/pod-product-compliance
Lightning Source LLC
Chambersburg PA
CBHW030429290526
45786CB00001B/204